At the Front
in a World War I
Field Hospital

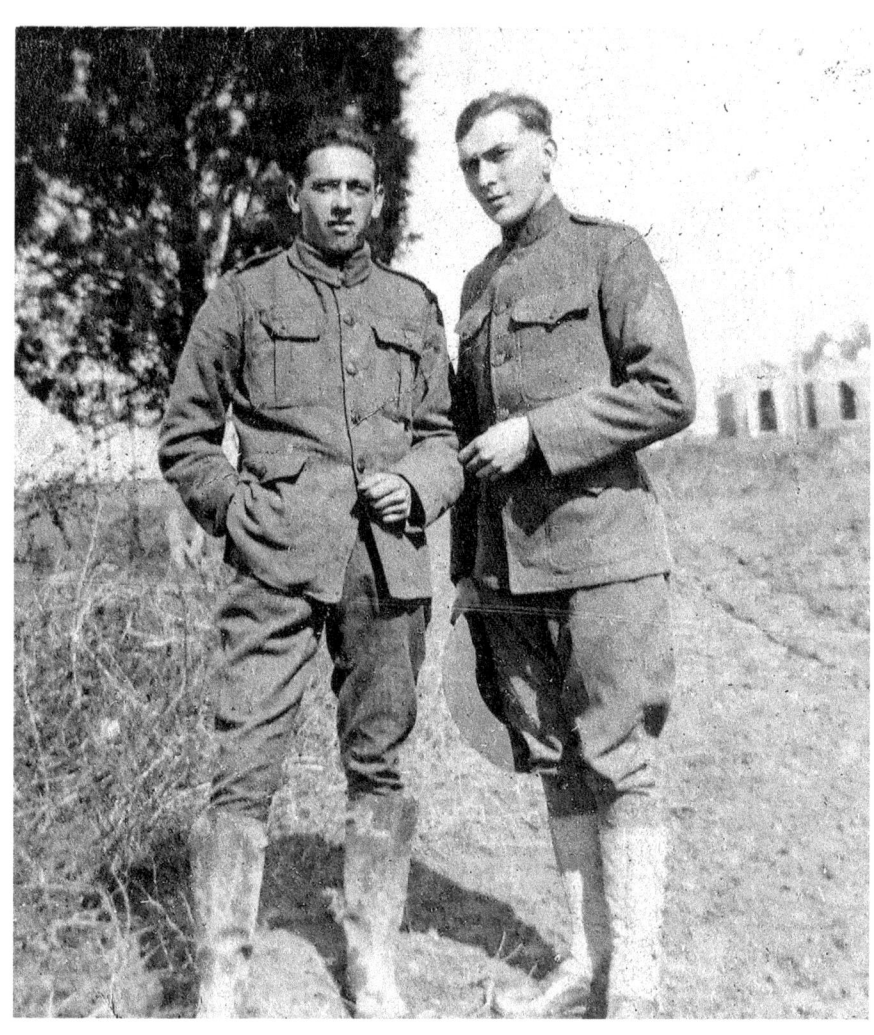

At the Front in a World War I Field Hospital

The Diaries and Letters of a 1st Sergeant in France

Leland N. Brown
Edited by Will Brown

Foreword by Thomas I. Faith

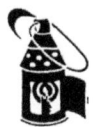

McFarland & Company, Inc., Publishers
Jefferson, North Carolina

Frontispiece: 1st Sergeant Brown (on right) with an unidentified fellow soldier at Camp Greene, North Carolina, around May of 1918 (photo album).

ISBN (print) 978-1-4766-7629-6
ISBN (ebook) 978-1-4766-5751-6

LIBRARY OF CONGRESS CATALOGING DATA ARE AVAILABLE

Library of Congress Control Number 2025026987

© 2025 Will Brown. All rights reserved

No part of this book may be reproduced or transmitted in any form or by any means, electronic or mechanical, including photocopying or recording, or by any information storage and retrieval system, without permission in writing from the publisher.

Front cover images: Sgt. Brown at the corner of 57th and Chester Avenue, Philadelphia, before he shipped overseas (photograph album); diary pages and book (author collection).

Printed in the United States of America

*McFarland & Company, Inc., Publishers
Box 611, Jefferson, North Carolina 28640
www.mcfarlandpub.com*

To the forgotten servicemen
and women
who served in World War I

Table of Contents

Acknowledgments — ix
Foreword by Thomas I. Faith — 1
Abbreviations and Glossary — 3
Preface — 5

Chapter 1. Camp Greene — 13
Chapter 2. At Sea — 40
Chapter 3. France — 46
Chapter 4. Gassed — 101
Chapter 5. Germany — 128

Afterword — 131
Appendix A: Training to Be a Soldier in the Medical Department in World War I — 145
Appendix B: The Personnel of Field Hospital No. 33 — 149
Bibliography — 225
Index — 227

Acknowledgments

I am grateful to a number of people who have helped me bring this book to fruition. I extend my thanks here. To Elizabeth McGuire of the Collingdale Historical Society, who enthusiastically supported this project from the beginning. To Elizabeth Widdicombe, who insisted that it should be published and made sure that it would be, by suggesting that McFarland would be a good fit. To the enthusiastic early readers of the manuscript who made useful suggestions: Ruth Fine, Margaret Kirk, George Marcus, and Leo Robinson. To the following archivists and librarians, who found what I needed: Megan McCall, of the Map Collection of the Free Library of Philadelphia; Caitlin Angelone, the reference librarian of the College of Physicians, Philadelphia; and Dan Flanagan, the alumni archivist of the Philadelphia College of the Sciences.

Ancestry.com and Newspapers.com were my main sources of genealogical and historic information about soldiers of Field Hospital No. 33 of the 4th Division. Through Ancestry.com records, I was able to contact the descendants of some of Sergeant Brown's fellow soldiers. To those who generously shared photographs and information about their World War I ancestors who had experiences similar to my father's during that bloody, senseless war: Lisa St. John, Jean Curran Meuli, Adrian Barkman, Jo Ann Zink Duprey, Laurie Miles, Bud Wilmerding, and Tina Miller. And a big "thank you" to Thomas I. Faith, who wrote the thoughtful foreword to this publication.

To my brother, Leland Blair Brown, who kept the diary safe until I could transcribe it and who voiced his insightful and clear remembrances of our father, and to his daughter Carolyn Taylor Brown, who photographed various memorabilia that Sergeant Brown had collected.

To my editor at McFarland, Layla Milholen, who supported my efforts and guided me with a gentle hand through the process.

To my best friend, my companion of 57 years, Emily Brown, for her patience, encouragement, and proofreading—and for the occasional much-needed kicks in the pants.

And, of course, most of all, to "Pop," whom I wish I could thank personally. He saw the importance of recording his experiences in a clear and personal manner and had the foresight and tenacity to write as much as he did. I wish he had felt free to write about it more openly. I very much wish he were here to enjoy this publication with us.

Thanks, Pop!

Foreword

Thomas I. Faith

The events experienced by doughboy Leland Nelson Brown were shared by many others in the United States Army during World War I. U.S. citizens collectively watched the rapid deterioration in United States–German relations following the reelection of President Woodrow Wilson in November 1916. In February 1917, the United States severed diplomatic relations with Germany over the conduct of unrestricted submarine warfare against commercial passenger ships, and in April the United States declared war on Germany following the public disclosure of the Zimmermann telegram, in which Germany discussed the possibility of forming a secret anti–U.S. alliance with Mexico. The Selective Service Act was passed in May to help raise the four million–man army the United States would train and equip for service overseas, and the first U.S. soldiers—including the commander of the American Expeditionary Forces, John J. Pershing—arrived in France in June.

Brown's experiences in enlistment and training were shared by many others. With 312,525 soldiers enlisted, the Commonwealth of Pennsylvania was second only to New York in World War I enlistees. The majority of U.S. soldiers in World War I had some formal schooling and could, like Brown, read and write in English, but roughly a quarter of them could not. As was typical of other well-educated professionals in the United States during World War I, Brown's professional training was not taken into account at his enlistment, and he became a private. He was sent to Camp Greene in North Carolina, which was home to more than 30,000 soldiers at that time, and assigned to serve with Field Hospital No. 33—one of four field hospital units in the newly constituted U.S. Army 4th Division.

When the 4th Division arrived in France between May and June in 1918, it was over a year after the United States formally entered the conflict, and almost four years after the war began in Europe in August 1914. After arriving, Brown and his fellow doughboys were equipped and trained as they commenced joint operations with the French military. During the Aisne-Marne operation in July, Field Hospital No. 33 was attached to the French triage and hospital for non-transportable wounded at Acy-en-Multien, then ordered east to Épaux-Bézu with Field Hospital No. 19 to operate a medical station for the seriously wounded and sick. In August all of the 4th Division's field hospital units were moved to a château near Fère-en-Tardenois, where they established a hospitalization center on the grounds. Field Hospital No. 33 continued to care for the sick and wounded of the 4th Division, rarely remaining in the same place for more than a few days, through the Saint-Mihiel and Meuse-Argonne operations until the Armistice on November 11, 1918, ended the fighting in Europe. The 4th Division suffered a total of 9,917 wounded soldiers and 2,903 deaths, after a total 47 days of frontline service.

Brown was one of 2,472 members of the 4th Division who were injured by gas. While the Army Medical Department, with 152,300 personnel, was one of the larger Army departments during World War I (third only to Infantry and Artillery), noncombatant service members experienced relatively few casualties. Fewer than 4,000 men in the Army Medical Department suffered injury or death over the course of the war out of the estimated 320,000 total U.S. casualties for World War I.

After the war, the headquarters of the 4th Division were assigned to Bad Bertrich, Germany. While they waited for transport home, the soldiers of the American Expeditionary Forces performed duties associated with the occupation of Germany, took regular leave to travel Europe, arranged a variety of sporting and gaming events, and attended classes on a variety of subjects both at schools in Europe and in educational programs organized by the Army. The 4th Division returned to the United States in July 1919, a little over a year after they had arrived in Europe.

Brown can be considered an "ordinary doughboy" in the sense that others who served the United States in uniform shared similar experiences to his during World War I. The curiosity and adventurous spirit reflected in his diary and letters, as well as his connection to family and longing for home, were feelings shared by many of his comrades overseas. Readers will no doubt agree, however, that the sacrifices and achievements made by Brown and the other members of his generation could never be described as ordinary.

Thomas I. Faith is a historian at the U.S. Department of State and the author of Behind the Gas Mask: The U.S. Chemical Warfare Service in War and Peace.

Abbreviations and Glossary

Abbreviations found in the diaries

A.E.F.	American Expeditionary Forces
A.N.C.	Army Nurse Corps
A.P.O.	Army Post Office
A.W.L.	Absent with leave
A.W.O.L.	Absent without leave
B.H.	Base Hospital
Bn.	Battalion
C.O.	Commanding Officer
E.H.	Evacuation Hospital
F.A.	Field Artillery
F.H.	Field Hospital
G.O.	General Orders
Hq.	Headquarters
M.O.T.C.	Medical Officers Training Camp
M.R.C.	Medical Reserve Corps
Q.M.C.	Quarter Master Corps
S.C.D.	Surgeon Certificate of Disability
S.O.	Standing Orders
S.O.S.	service of supply
S.U.	Staging Unit

Glossary

ammunition train—a fleet of wagons or trucks carrying munitions

balling the jack—going as fast as one can

billet—quarters assigned by a military order to soldiers in a private home or a structure where soldiers stay

Boche—a derogatory term given to the Germans by the French; Loosely translated, it means "pigheaded."

Bulletin—*The Philadelphia Evening Bulletin*, a newspaper

casual—a soldier that was a temporary member of a company

casual company— a company of soldiers who are in transit

Dutch—a bastardization of the word "Deutsch," as the Germans call themselves

Inquirer—*The Philadelphia Inquirer*, a newspaper

noncom—a noncommissioned soldier with the rank from corporal through sergeant

Record—*The Philadelphia Record*, a newspaper

Sanitary Train—the division of the army responsible for the health of the soldier; it included the field, evacuations, and base hospitals as well as ambulance companies.

service of supply—the division of the army responsible for supplies and material to support the army

Preface

Leland Brown, my father, kept a diary while in the Army during World War I. My brother, Lee, remembers knowing of the diary's existence while my father was living, but it was never brought out to be read or discussed. After "Pop" died in 1984 at age 90, the diary was passed down and finally came to me about eight years ago. In the fall of 2016, I decided to transcribe it.

I have tried to do so as faithfully as possible. Some punctuation has been corrected to make it more readable. My father had a penchant in the diaries for capitalizing words excessively, and this I did not alter. He also did not use accents in names of individuals or places and sometimes used abbreviations for months rather than spelling them out. I did not add accents or spell out the months in my transcription. I've included some of the images and clippings found within the diary and have added a few more.

There are several places where he used racial slurs to describe Black persons. He is responsible for using those words, but I found them so abhorrent to read that I substituted the word "Black" for the words he used.

Leland started a photo album while he was in his advanced training at Camp Greene, North Carolina. Images from that album bear a "photo album" notation. In a letter home, he asked his parents to take good care of it, indicating that he had not taken the album overseas with him. Some photos seem to have been placed in the album on his return to the United States. These have a certain patina that suggests they were carried loosely through the rigors of the war.

While transcribing the diary I remembered that there were letters he had written to his family that were then faithfully transcribed into composition books by his parents. Often the letters and diary describe the same events, told differently. My first thought was to edit out redundant material from the letters home, but, since the way in which he wrote the letters varies from the diary, I decided to include them in their totality. The letters are shown in italics.

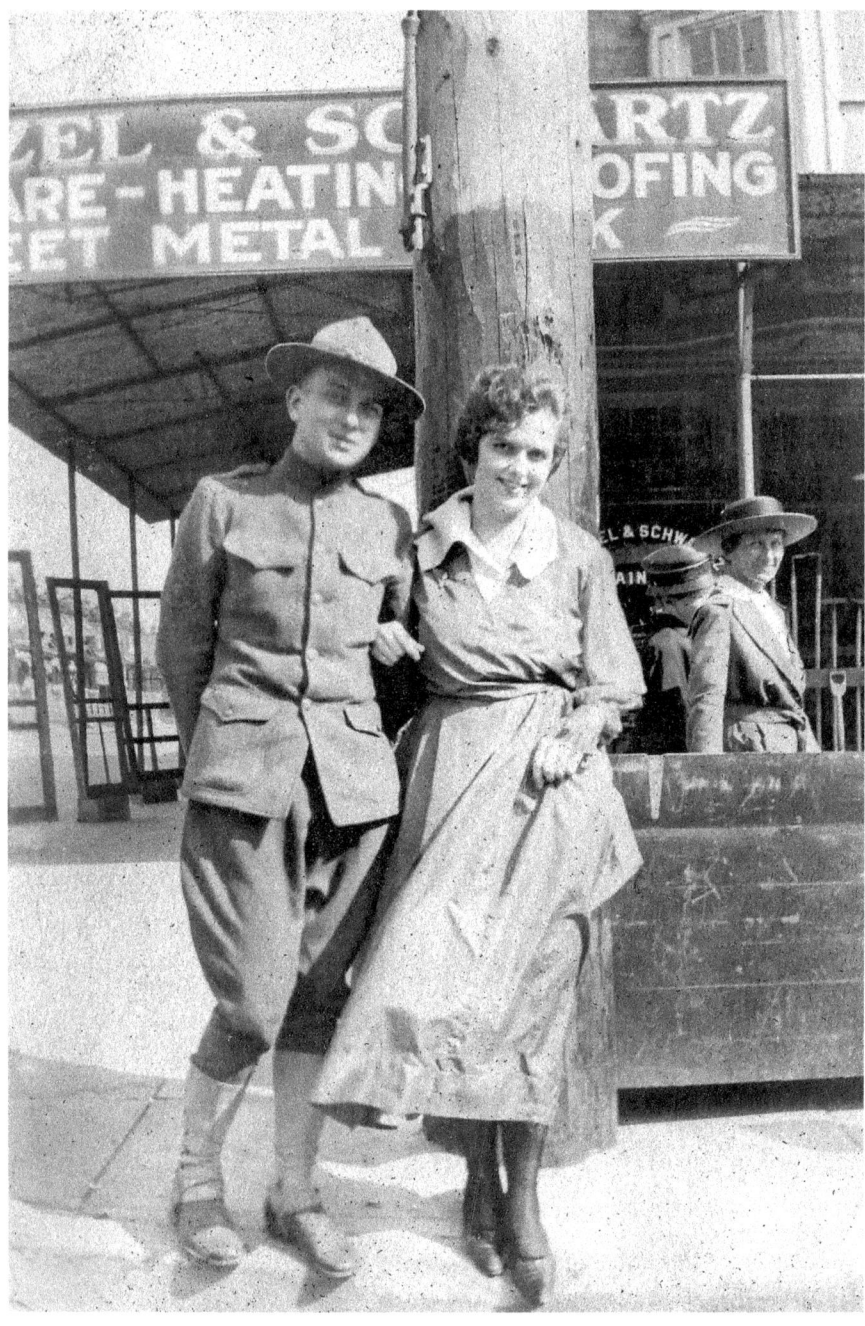

Sergeant Brown with his girlfriend, Marian, at the corner of 57th Street and Chester Avenue, Philadelphia, before he shipped overseas (photo album).

Reading his letters and diary entries and pursuing information relating to his writings about the war gave me a better understanding of a time about which I had known very little. It had seemed only a foggy chapter in world history, long before I was born.

* * * * *

Leland Nelson Brown was born on October 20, 1893, in Smyrna, Delaware, to William F. Brown, a tailor, and his wife, Nora West Cotton. He was the first of their three children—all sons. Both parents descended from families that had been on the Delmarva Peninsula since the early 1700s, mostly as farmers or, in the case of his mother's family, carriage makers and dry goods merchants as well as farmers. Some of their families prospered earlier, but whatever wealth they had obtained had dissipated by the time Nora and William married. Neither of Leland's parents went beyond the eighth grade in their schooling. His father, William (Will), was a tailor who had probably apprenticed in that trade with his future father-in-law, Harry Cotton.

Will's partnership in the tailoring business in Smyrna fell apart when his partner took all the assets and left him with the outstanding accounts payable. It was about this time that the family moved to the Kensington area of Philadelphia so that Will would have a better chance of finding employment as a tailor.

Leland attended public schools and graduated in 1911 from Northeast Manual Training School for Boys in Philadelphia. Later that year the family moved to Collingdale, Pennsylvania, a suburb of Philadelphia.

His first job after high school was with an electrical supply company on Chestnut Street, Philadelphia. In 1913 he found employment as a clerk in a drugstore in Darby, Pennsylvania, and, later in that year, he worked in a drugstore in West Philadelphia owned by Harry B. Holland. Holland was childless and took a liking to Leland, perhaps seeing him as the son he never had. Holland encouraged him to attend the Philadelphia College of Pharmacy (now the University of the Sciences), acting as his preceptor. How his tuition was paid is unknown, but certainly his parents were in no financial condition to cover it. It is thought that Holland may have undertaken that responsibility or that Leland was able to pay for it out of his salary. He did work for Holland while he was in college. In June 1917 he was awarded a Doctor of Pharmacy degree. The subject of his senior thesis was "Cannabis—Its Cultivation."

Germany invaded France in 1914, but the United States did not enter the war until April 1917. Leland probably had a commitment to Harry Holland and worked with him until his sense of patriotism and peer pressure overcame him. Or perhaps he was worried about being drafted. If drafted, he wouldn't be able to choose which service he would be attached to, or to what branch of a service he would be assigned. If he enlisted, he would have that choice. It is assumed he initially signed up at the recruiting office

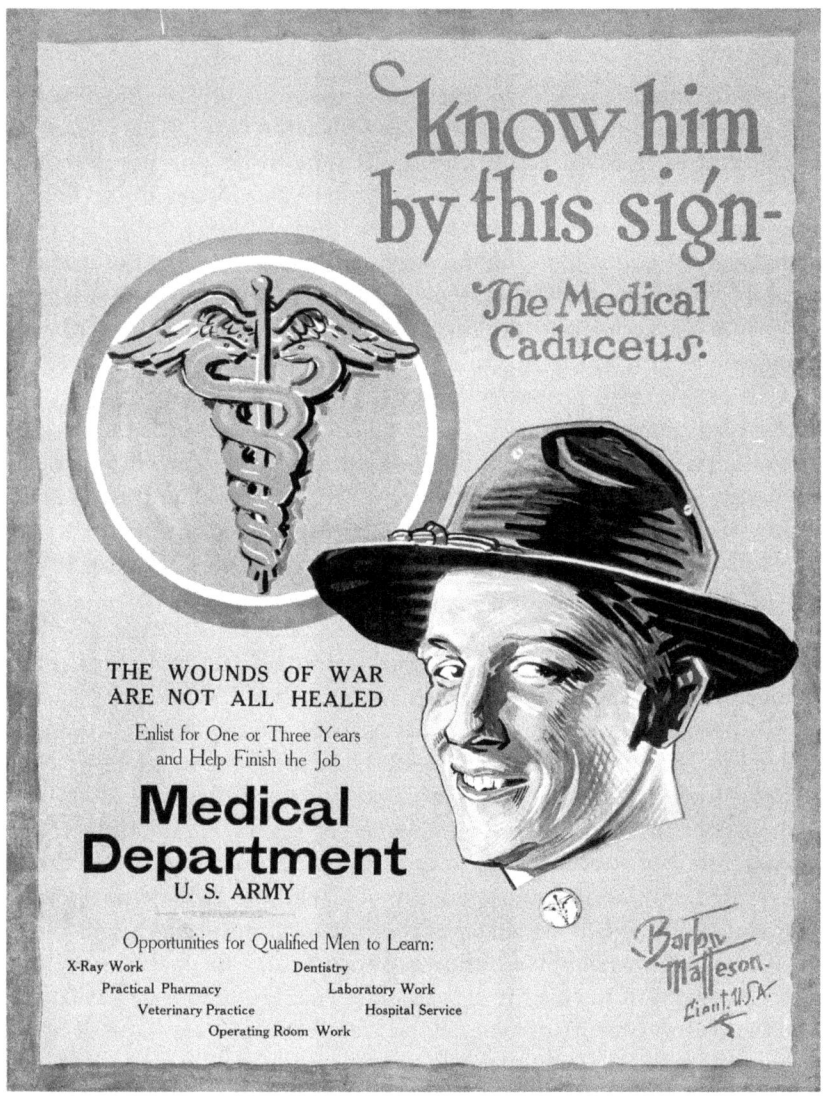

World War I recruitment poster for the Army Medical Department. The poster states that one may enlist for one or three years and promises "Opportunities for Qualified Men to Learn: X-Ray Work, Practical Pharmacy, Veterinary Practice, Operating Room Work, Dentistry, Laboratory Work [and] Hospital Service" (Library of Congress). http://www.loc.gov/pictures/item/00651835/.

at 1229 Arch Street in Philadelphia. He was then sent to Fort Slocum, New York, where he was subject to a physical examination. If he passed the physical, he would be in the Army. He did pass, and he chose the Medical Department.

Leland received his basic training at Medical Officers Training Corps at Camp Greenleaf, Fort Oglethorpe, Georgia. His advanced training was at Camp Greene, North Carolina, where his diary begins.

He wrote in the first pages of the second volume of the diary the following:

> I have often thought of my grandmother's brother, who fought in the Civil War. I remember very plainly the thrills I had when I read the diary which he kept in 1863. I remember how I used to wish that he would have been more fuller in his explanations of his experiences. I hope that I may write a full story of my part over here so that I may refresh my memory as soon as I get home.

His outfit was the 4th Division and his company was Field Hospital No. 33, which was part of the all-encompassing medical unit—the Sanitary Train. The Sanitary Train was the unit that supported the entire division's health needs. This served not only the wounded and sick, but those suffering from shell shock, skin and venereal diseases, and psychological trauma.

The Sanitary Train at the front consisted of several layers of organization. The closest to the front were the litter bearers, who brought the wounded or gassed from the battlefield to the awaiting ambulances. The ambulances brought the wounded to a field hospital that was close to the front lines, usually within six to eight miles from the front. The field hospital would serve as a dressing station or a triage. This is where Sergeant Brown worked. The cases would be sorted out by severity of their wounds. Their wounds would be dressed, and, if they were severe enough, the patient would be transferred to an evacuation hospital where further treatment such as surgery or the splinting of limbs would be carried out. Surgery could also happen at a field hospital. The evacuation hospital would, ideally, be located further behind the front lines than the field hospital and adjacent to a railroad in order to facilitate transfer to a base hospital if the soldier needed extended treatment. Adjacent field hospitals would often have separate functions—such as triage or treating the sick, gassed, or seriously wounded. Even though field hospitals were not usually directly on the front line, they were subject to artillery (both by gas and conventional shells) and aerial bombing. Once at a base hospital, the patient would receive additional treatment and recuperate before returning to duty or returning to the United States.

It appears that Leland's degree as a pharmacist was not taken into account when he became a soldier. The Army did not give pharmacists commissions as officers as they did other medical personnel—dental, veterinary, and medical doctors. It was suggested by the American Pharmaceutical Association that qualified pharmacists be granted a commission, but Congress never enacted the necessary legislation to do so. If the legislation had passed, it would have required graduate pharmacists to have at least five years of experience as a pharmacist. Evidently this was resented by qualified pharmacists, although there is no mention of this by Leland. He entered the Army as a buck private on October 2, 1917. He was promoted to private first class three months later and sergeant one month after that; finally he became a sergeant first class two and a half months after he was made sergeant. His degree in pharmacy may account for his quick rise as a first sergeant, although his duties at the field hospital appear not to have had anything to do with his pharmaceutical expertise. There may have been other contributing factors, such as his dedication to the Army's cause and his hard work. There were three privates in his outfit who attained the rank of sergeant first class who were in a medical field before enlistment: Steven Lombard, Leland Brown, and Arthur Fisher. Lombard was a mortician, while Brown and Fisher were pharmacists.

In the beginning of the diary, Leland is merely recording the day-to-day events at the field hospital at Camp Greene. Later on, he opens up and describes his experiences in greater detail and his writing becomes more interesting.

While reading his letters and diary entries, one has little sense of what sort of work he was doing. One of his letters home indicates that his parents were also not informed of what he did. He responds to their query:

> My work is just the same as it was in the states. I look out for the records. I have two separate departments—1st the hospital with patients and 2nd the company. I have two separate shifts.… My work is overseeing. I do not do much work with my hands. I say yes or no or do it this way or that way.

He also would maintain records of the patients being admitted and forward that information on to Washington so that families could be notified.

Reading his diary has given me a new understanding of my father. There is so much that he described, yet I wonder how much he left out. He did talk about his experiences with us during his service, but not very often and in little detail. There are so many questions I wish I had asked him about it while he was still living.

Will Brown, October 2025

Leland wrote home from Fort Slocum, New York, describing the experiences of his enlistment:

Preface

Sept. 2, 1917
Tuesday—Noon

Dear Folks-

Just had dinner. Arrived safe here last night. Did not get to go to bed until after midnight. Then only for a few hours sleep. Was up at 5 A.M. and had breakfast. Then marched all over camp to be examined. Had no trouble passing. They sure did make it emphatic that drafted men could not enlist. Hope I have not received any notice. If I have please send me word when it came as I want to start to tell these people here about it. Everything is fine. Breakfast we had all we could eat. Sausage Bread—no butter, coffee with sugar and milk—Potatoes Boiled.

Dinner—

Coffee-Baked Beans, cake, Rice & Potatoes

I have been vaccinated for small pox & inoculated against typhoid. The typhoid makes me feel a little light headed but I am ok every other way. I am afraid that I ate too much for dinner.

Write and let me know about the draft business as I am anxious about it. Saw Dr. Roddy this morning. Did not get a chance to talk to him, but will as soon as I have time. We are out on Long Island Sound about 18 or 20 miles from New York. We came to New Rochelle and then the trolly to Fort Slocum wharf and then out on the boat to the island on which Fort Slocum is located.

I will write more tomorrow when I get over this typhoid inoculation.

Me—

Chapter 1

CAMP GREENE

[Beginning of Diary]

H. 2. Sanitary Unit Bn. #6.

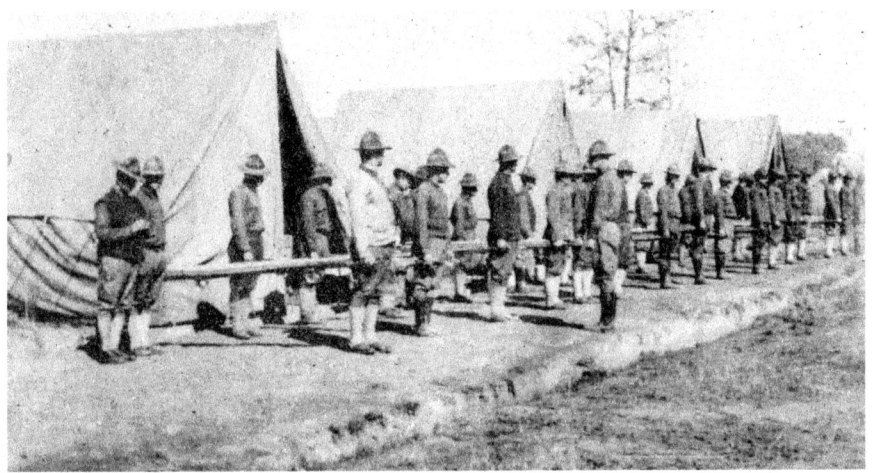

Inspection at Camp Greene (photo album).

1917

November 1, 1917

Provisional field hospital "G" organized per par. #1 G.O. #3 Medical officers assigned for duty.

1st Lt. F.P. Fitzpatrick M.R.C. Commanding officer.

1st Lts. Leo F. Tarkington, M.R.C., Edw. Pitcairn M.R.C., Iris J. Slay M.R.C., Arthur Hartley M.R.C. per. II #2

Sgts. Smithy, Brady, Hoyt, Meyers, Gould, Hodson [Hodsdon] per par. 3.

Thirty six privates per par #3.

Pvt. C.M. Hickerson assigned from F.H. 23 per par 2 S.O. #37, Hg. S.U. Bn #6.

November 2

Sgt. Carlos Mena joined for duty per par #2 S.O. #4 Hg. S.U. Bn. #4

Pvt. Chas W. Preston assigned per par #5 S.O. #4 Hg. S.U. Bn #6

Pvt. Bryan J. Dickinson transferred to F.H. 23 per par #2 S.O. #40 F.H. Hg. Nov. 2, 17.

November 3

Inspection 9 am by Maj. Weiser.

Nov. 4

Pvt. Evans reported by officer of [the] Day—J. Peters—"Smoking in Stables." Confined to Company streets for 12 days commencing Nov. 5/17 to Nov. 17/17.

Nov. 5

Private Hickerson returned today fr. sick in hospital Nov. 5/17

Nov. 6/17

Articles of war, rules and regulations read to the Co. Nov. 6/17. Pvt. Oscar Cato transferred to F.H. # 23 per. Par. #1 S.O. 41 FH. Hq. Nov. 6/17. Pvt Peters trans. to F.H. G from F.H. 23 per. Par.#2 S.O. 41 F.H. Hg Nov. 6/17

Nov. 8/17

Pvt. Preston confined to the limits of Company streets for [2] weeks for disrespect to non. Com. Officers. Nov. 8/17 to Nov. 22/17

Nov. 10/17

Pvt. Myrkle discharged Nov. 10/17 physical disability

Nov. 12/17

1st Lt. Pitcairn relieved from further duty with F.H. "G." Nov. 11/17

Nov. 13/17

Pvt. Charles Bossert A.W.O.L.

Nov. 14/17

Field Hospital "G" designated Field Hospital No. 33 effective Nov. 13th 1917

Nov. 15/17

Pvt. Havey & Pvt. Phillips A.W.O.L. from Reville [sic] Nov. 15 Returned by Provost Guard 10:00 A.M. sd. Charges to be preferred by Provost Marshall. Pvt. Hancock sent to Hospital.

Nov. 17/17

4 Pvts joined for duty from Sanitary Co. #1 Camp Greenleaf Post Fort Oglethorpe Ga. Per. V.O. Director Field Hospitals

Nov. 17/17

Pvt. Moore Henry from sick in Hospital to duty. Pvt. Harvey Edwards from A.W.O.L. to confinement.

Nov. 19

1st Lieut. Humphries N. Ervin M.R.C. joined for duty Nov. 18/17 from Btln. #4 Post per par. 5 S.O. 172 Nov. 16, 1917 Hg. Camp Greenleaf.

Nov. 20/17

Pvt. Charles Bossert from A.W.O.L. to confinement Nov. 20/17

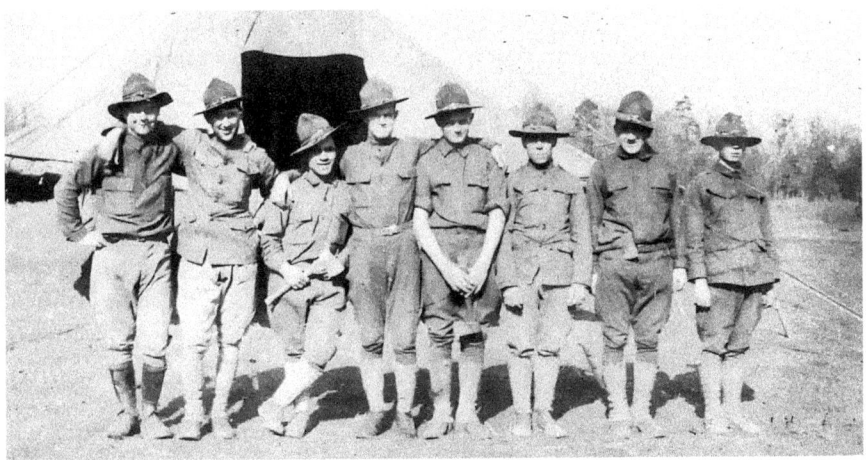

Fellow soldiers from Field Hospital No. 33 at Camp Greene, North Carolina (photo album).

Nov 23/17

Pvt. Harvey Edwards from confinement to punishment given by Company Commander for a period of 10 days.

Nov. 24/17

Pvts. Booth, Plemon, Brown, M. Sirikel one week company punishment & one week confinement Nov. 24 to Dec 7. The following named men are confined to company streets for one week Nov. 24/17 to Dec 1/17 Claycourt, Parkhurst, Marchand, Fisher, Cooper, Brown L., Kohlman.

Nov. 25/17

Pvt. Joseph Plummet from duty to sick in Hospital

Nov. 26/17

1st Lieut. Walter Dick. M.R.C. joined for duty Nov. 25/17 per. par. 4 S.O. 5, Hg. Bn H. post sd. Pvts, George Ward & William Bishop, joined for duty Nov. 25/17 per par. 1 S.O. 50 Hg. F.H. Jost. sd. Pvts. Luther S. Plemons, Irving Booth, Cecil R. Eddington, Francis Hommes, Dewey W. Jones, Harry Kohman, George H. Schreiber, James H. Schuhl, trans to F.H. #25 per. Par. 2, S.O. 50, Hg. Field Hospital Camp Greenleaf, Ft. Oglethorpe, Ga.

Dec 13

Pvt. James C. Burt fr. duty to sick in hospital p. p. 1st ind. Hg. Camp Surgeon, Camp Greene, Charlotte N.C.

Pvts. John Y. Biddle, Phillip Enwright, Bernard Garbrock, Ernest Huekls, Thomas E. Jordan, Peter Lista, Thomas F. McDonwell (German Measles Contact cases) from duty to Detention Camp p. p. 2 ,1st ind. Hg. Camp Surgeon Camp Greene, Charolette, N.C., Dec. 2, 1917. Private Stephen Green fr. duty to abs. without leave per memo. Hg. Camp Greene, Charlotte, N.C., Dec 8, 1917.

Dec 15

Pvts. Albert Frederick, Stephen Greene, Daniel L. Dixon appointed cooks. Private William W. Havey [Haney], Murice DeWalt, Peter Fast, George E. Hall, Phillip H. Lawrence, James J. Mullaney, Oscar H. Miner from duty to abs. without leave per memo Hg. Camp Greene, N.C. Dec. 8, 1917.

Dec 20

Cook Stephen Greene from A.W.O.L. to duty. Sgt. Martin E. Hoyt

Jr. from duty to A.W.L. Pvt. Edgar R. Grimm from duty to Hospital. Pvt. Edw. F. Quinn from duty to sick in quarters.

Dec 21

Pvt. Maurice DeWalt from A.W.L. to duty. Pvt. Edw. F. Quinn fr. sick in quarters to hospital. Pvts. Philip Kersky and Charles J. Soldo from duty to confinement.

Dec 22

Pvt. Peter Fast from A.W.L. to duty.

Dec 23

Pvts. George E Hall and Philip H. Lawrence from A.W.L. to duty. 1st Lieutenants Walter Dick and Francis B. Ring from duty to A.W.L. Privates William W. Haney, James J. Mullaney and Oscar H. Miner from A.W.L. to A.W.O.L. Privates John H. Page, George Zinc [Zink], Howard G. Scheidle and Tom L. Stewart from duty to A.W.L.

Dec 24

1st Lieut I.J. Slay fr. duty to abs. with leave. Pvts. William W. Haney, James J. Mullaney and Oscar H. Miner from A.W.O.L. to arrest.

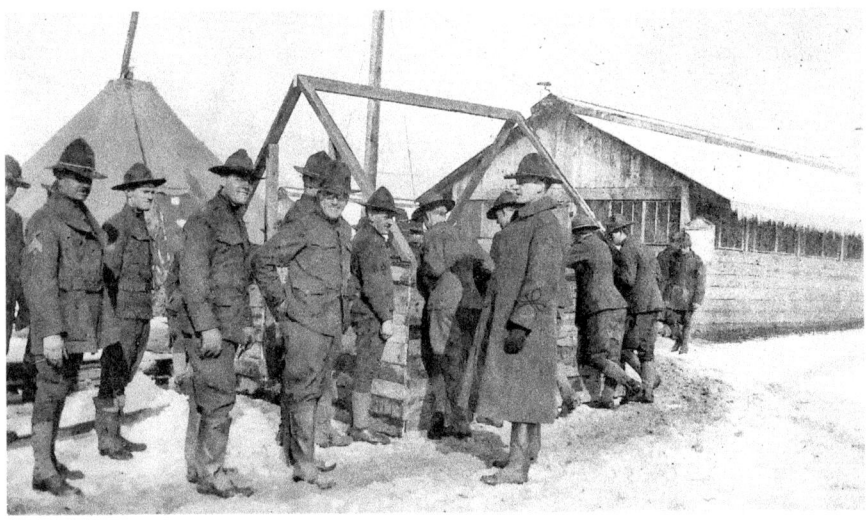

At Camp Greene, North Carolina. Moving the officers tent. The officer wearing the overcoat is probably Lieutenant Francis Fitzpatrick, and the sergeant on the left is most likely Sergeant First Class Carlos Mena (photo album).

Dec 26

Pvt. James C. Burt fr. hospital to duty. Pvts. Oscar H. Miner and James J. Mullaney from arrest to duty.

Dec. 28

Pvts. J.Y. Biddle, Phillip Enwright, Brernard Garbrock, Ernest Huekles, Thomas E. Jordan, Peter Lista, and Thomas McDonnell, German Measels contact cases from detention Camp to duty.

Pvts. Lawrence D. King and Fred P. Eberle fr. duty to abs with leave.

Pvt. George Zinc [Zink] from abs with leave to duty.

Pvt. Howard G. Scheidle fr abs with leave to A.W.O.L.

Dec. 29

1st Lieut. Francis P. Fitzpatrick, C.O. appointed Captain M.R.C. Commission dated December 14, 1917.

Pvt. Howard G Scheidle from A.W.O.L. to arrest.

Dec. 30

Sgt. Martin E. Hoyt Jr. from abs. with leave to duty.

Pvt. Frank Borowsky fr duty to abs. with leave.

Pvt. Howard H. Scheidle from arrest to duty.

Dec 31

Pvts. Tom L. Stewart and John H. Page fr. abs. with leave to duty.

Pvts. Thomas J. Burns, Leland N. Brown and Edward W. Hind fr. duty to abs. with leave.

Pvt. James J. Mullaney fr. duty to A.W.O.L.

1918

Jan. 1

Pvt. James J. Mullaney fr. A.W.O.L. to arrest.

Jan 3

1st Lieut Walter Dick, 1st Lieut James B. Ring, 1st Lieut Iris J. Slay fr. abs with leave to duty.

Chapter 1. Camp Greene

Jan 4

Pvt. James J. Mullaney fr. arrest to confinement. Pvt. Philip H. Lawrence fr. duty to arrest. Pvt. Heber D. Gregg from duty to special duty at Divisional Statistical Office.

Jan 5

Pvt. Lawrence D. King fr. abs. with leave to duty.

Received two mules, harness and escort wagon by requisition fr. Quartermaster.

Jan 6

Pvt. Leland N. Brown fr abs. with leave to duty.

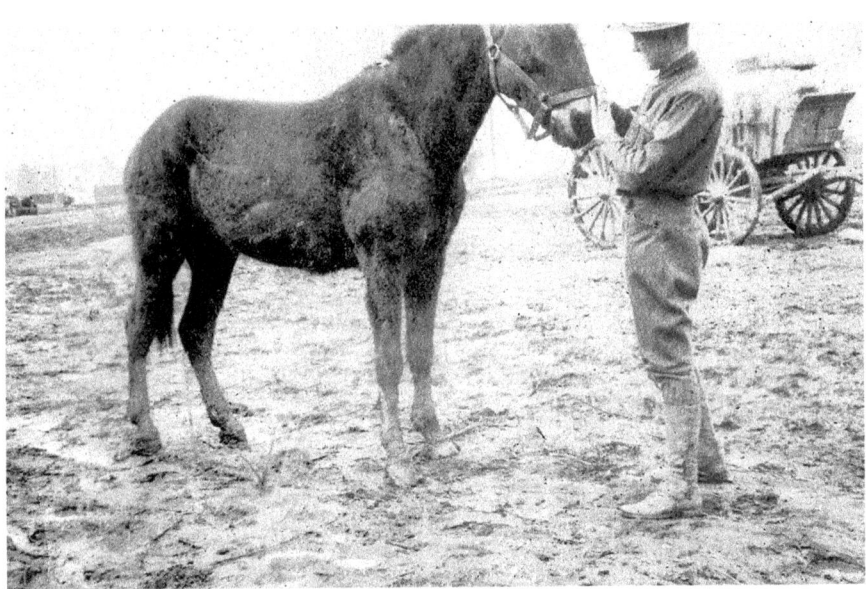

An Army mule with an escort wagon at Camp Greene. This could be Private Sadowski, who tended the mules. See the diary entry of March 16, 1918, which mentions Private Sadowski and the mules (photo album).

Jan. 7

Pvt. Edw. F. Quinn fr. hospital to duty. Pvts. Thomas J. Burns, Fred P. Eberle and Frank Borowsky fr. abs. with leave to duty.

Pvt. Phillip H. Lawrence fr. arrest to duty.

1st Lieut Francis B. Ring on special duty with Regimental Infirmaries, Fourth Division.

Jan. 8
Pvt. Edward W. Hind fr. abs. with leave to duty.

Jan. 9
Pvt. James J. Mullaney fr. confinement to duty.

Jan. 10. Thursday
One sergeant and two privates attached for rations fr. Hg. Director of Field Hospital Company Jan. 8, 1917 at 11:30 A.M.

Jan. 1–10th
Station & Record of Events Camp Greene, Charlotte, N.C.
Usual Camp Duties.

January 12. Saturday
Pvt. Phillip H. Kersky fr. confinement to duty.

Pvt. LeRoy Shearer fr. duty to A.W.O.L.

Pvt. Edward F. Quinn "Discharged." per S.C.D. 4th Ind. Hg. Camp Greene, N.C. Jan. 8, 1918. Service honest and Faithful Character "Excellent."

January 13
Pvt. John Garden A.W.O. L.

January 16
Received news that a bunch of the boys were appointed privates first. Here is the list. Jess B. Bowman, Leland N. Brown, Arthur R. Fisher, Bernard Garbrock, Andrew Youngblood [Jongbloed], Lawrence D. King, Stephen S. Lombard, James J. Mullaney, Roy Shearer, John S. Whitney, Walter R. Wise, George Zinc [Zink], John S. Broxterman, Thomas J. Burns, James C. Burt, James J. Carlin, Guy R. Daniel, Fred P. Eberly, Peter Fast, Don G. Gorham, William W. Havey [Haney], Carlton M. Hickerson, Edward W. Hind, Peter Lista, John H. Page, Arthur L. Phillips, Charles J. Soldo, Tom L. Stewart, Alexander I. Szczypin, Alfredo Trenta, Richard J. Zipse.

The authority of their appointment was 1st Ind off. Div Surg. 4th Dic (Reg) Camp Greene, Charlotte N. C., Jan. 14, 1918.

The boys sure were happy and who can blame them. The letter which contain these names was written about a month ago. Then Shearer and Soldo were in good standing but now Capt. Fitzpatrick wants them reduced so he has written to the Division Surgeon to have them reduced.

Privates Biddle, Hubles, Paquette, Perkins, Rubley and Spang were sent down to the Infirmary at the 16th Field Artillery to get some practical dope on hospital work.

January 17

Cook Stephen Green was reduced to grade of private because the table of organization does not allow us to have two cooks. I was talking to Green about it and he said that when he joined the Army he did it because he thought he couldn't get fired but now he sees that the army is the same as any other place.

January 18

We received a telegram last night from Fred W. Kottcamp, Chief of Police, York, Pa. and that he has arrested Shearer and a Private from some machine gun Battalion. They were arrested for stealing an automobile. The captain wired Kottcamp to send him back under guard.

The letter came back from the Division Surgeon that Shearer and Soldo had been reduced to Privates again. Dewalt, Gregg & Rizzo were made Privates First Class by the Division Surgeon, Lt. Col. Carswell, M.C. U.S.A.

January 20

Pvt. Grimm returned from the base hospital. He has tuberculosis. He is waiting for his discharge.

January 22

Lt. Ring came back to duty with the company.

January 23

Pvt. Grimer was Honorably Discharged today. Pvt. John Garden came back and reported to duty [and] the captain promptly slapped him the guard house. Shearer was reported as being in the guard house at Fort Howard, Maryland. Lt. William W. Jones M.C. and Lt. John R. Hall M.C. were assigned to this outfit for duty. Lt. Jones reported for duty.

January 24

Lieut. Hall reported for duty.

January 25

Pvt. Frank J. Nyakowski reported sick. Suspected that he has Cerebro-Spinal Meningitis. He was sent to the base hospital. We were all examined to see if we have any in us but all the reports were negative.[1]

---

1. During January and February of 1918 there was an epidemic of cerebrospinal meningitis at Camp Greene resulting in a number of deaths.

January 26

Acting Sgt. King went up the guardhouse and had Soldo taken out. Soldo is a bad egg. His trip to the "can" hasn't done him a bit of good, in fact, he is more defiant than ever.

January 28, 1918

Lieut. Jones is relieved from duty with Company yesterday. Pvt. William J. Sutton was arrested yesterday. I was getting ready to have a day off when they brought this old fake up here to the office. He cut his hand with a razor one day last month and it has never healed. He has been going around here throwing the bluff that he was sick. Well they have a goods on him now. Pvt. Lombard heard that he has been drinking a mixture of soap and water to make himself sick and he tried to buy croton oil but couldn't.[2] Then he bought some caustic and applied it to the cut on his hand to make it fester. Today they found a stick of shaving soap and a couple of pieces of caustic. The soap had the imprints of his teeth. He is a good for nothing man and should be punished accordingly.

A. R. Fisher, L.D. King, F.R. Eberly, Thomas McDonnell, Lombard, & Daniel were sent to the Base Hospital for special training. Fisher & Daniel are to learn how to administer ether & chloroform.

January 30

Six new recruits were assigned to the company. They came out from Fort Oglethorpe, Georgia. Their names are Fred Henning, Wilbur W. Frankfort, Carmen C. Delo, Victor A. Shock, Leon H. Walter, Allen Cole.

February 1, 1918

Pvt. Eddie Hind was appointed mechanic today. He is a good man and "knows all their is to know about autos."

February 2

Sgt. Mena and Pvts. Bowman and Garbrock went to the rifle range to learn how to shoot.

February 3

Pvts. Rubley, Perkins, Biddle, Hubles, Paquette & Spang came back from the 16th Field Artillery last night.

---

2. Croton oil taken internally in small doses can cause diarrhea. Externally, the oil can cause irritation and swelling.

Chapter 1. Camp Greene

February 4

Private Spang came up to the office today with his belly swelled up like a woman in a family way. He was operated on for appendicitis about six months ago and either the surgeon left the scissors in there or else he never took the appendix out. Spang was sent to the Base Hospital.

February 5

Mena, Bowman and Garbrock came home today. They had a swell time. Garbrock is the best shooter then Mena and Bowman is rotten.

February 6

Lieut. Ring removed some ingrowing toe nails for Pvt. Arthur L. Phillips. He has some sore foot.

February 9

Phillips was given a 10 day furlough and allowed to go to his home in Fort Wayne, Ind. He left last night at 8 o'clock.

February 11

Eberly, Enwright, King, Lombard and McDonnell came back from the Base Hospital and Cooper, Derrick, Garbrock, Rizzo and Schimska took their places. Lt. Herring thinks that Pvt. Perkins has the "cou" and he sent him to the Base Hospital for observation.

February 12

Private Green was sent to the hospital today. He has La grippe or influenza. Mearle [Merle] E. Hodsdon was appointed first sergeant to succeed Sgt. Mena.

February 14

Lt Hale [Hall] was relieved from duty with the company. He is C.O. of San. Squad #1, 4th Div (Reg).

February 15

Pvt. Philip Kersky was discharged today for minority concealed at enlistment.[3] He is a Jew from Philadelphia and has no money. The government refused to pay his transportation home.

---

3. "Minority concealed at enlistment" was researched, and no explanation was forthcoming. Perhaps if one made a false statement when enlisting, such as claiming to be of a different religion than one actually was, or if one were under- or overage, that would be enough for dismissal. Jews were certainly allowed to enlist in the Army.

February 16

Kersky has no money so the boys took up a collection [of] about $40 and gave it to him. Sgt. Hoyt bought him some clothes and a railroad ticket. Broxterman came back from the hospital today.

February 17

Lieut. William W. Jones, M.C. is assigned to this outfit again.

February 18

Arthur L. Phillips came back from his furlough today. The folks all gave him the glad hand when he was home and he was glad to get back with the boys.

February 19

The warrants arrived yesterday for the new Sergeants first class and the new Sergeants.

Sgt. Carlos Mena Jr and Mearle [Merle] E. Hodsdon were appointed Sgts. First Class and Jess B. Bowman, Leland N. Brown, Arthur R. Fisher, Andrew Jongbloed, Stephen S. Lombard and Albert Frederick were appointed Sergeants to rank from February 15.

Capt. Fitzpatrick presented the warrants. As the men's names were called they stepped up to the captain and saluted. Received the warrant, saluted again, did an about face and walked off. Frederick forgot the about-face and Brown forgot the second salute.

Matthew Brown, Haney and Edwards dissappeared [sic] today. No one knows where they have gone.

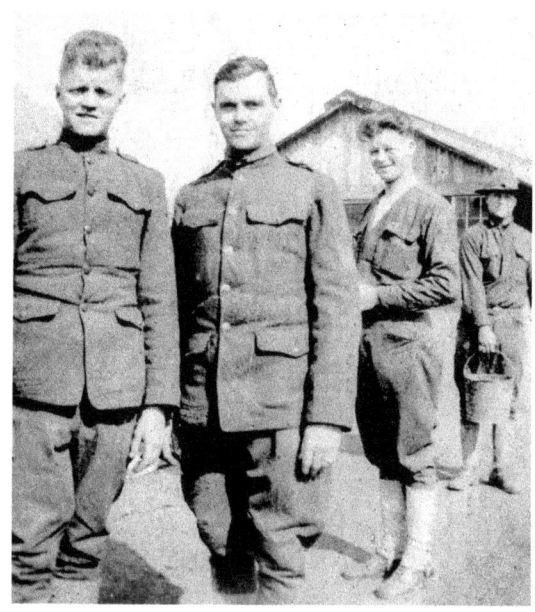

Sergeants Andrew Jongbloed, Stephen S. Lombard, and Jess B. Bowman, with Private Raymond J. Cooper (photo album).

February 20

M. Brown, Haney & Edwards were pinched by the Provost Guard at Gastonia, N.C. and were returned to duty today. They were all tried by S.C. and sentenced to pay a fine of ten days pay.

February 22

Lt. Johnson was sent to special duty at Casual Camp #1, Camp Greene, N.C. He took private Martin Anderson with him as orderly. Privates Lawrence D. King and Bernard Garbrock left here today as the Medical Detachment accompanying the 4th Div. Supply Train which is going to Buffalo N.Y.

Captain Fitz and Lieut. Dick left on a pass tonight. Destination unknown. Boy oh boy there will be a hot time in the old town tonight.

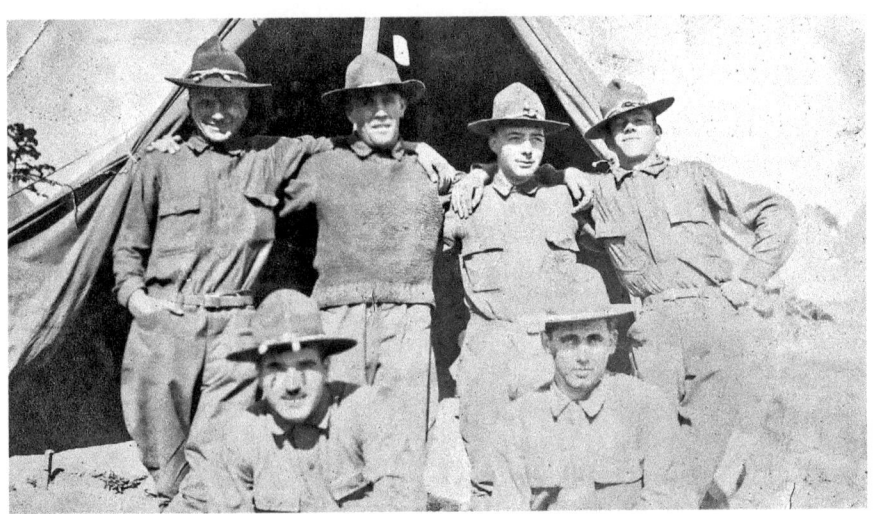

Buddies at Camp Greene: Lieutenant Francis P. Fitzpatrick in the sweater and Peter Lista in the back row on the far right. The other soldiers are unidentified (photo album).

February 24

Capt. Fitz & Lt. Dick arrived back this afternoon pretty much the worst for fair wear and tear in the service of the United States. Boys there must have been some hot rails between here and Washington according to the talk at the officers mess.

February 25

Lieut. Ring received orders to report to the Army Medical School,

Washington, D.C. March 4. He wrote to Gen. Cameron for a six day pass.

February 27

Lieut. Ring's pass arrived and he left last night.

February 28

The Co. went on a hike today. Sure did have a good time.

March 1

Private Enwright came back from his French leave.[4] Ready to take his medicine. He was put in the guardhouse.

March 2, 1918

Inspection today. Pretty good. It sure is hot weather. Tom Stewart was appointed Cook fr. Pvt. 1st class to take effect March 1, 1918. Tom sure is a funny fellow. He was born in the country famous for its moonshine. That's how Tom came to join the army. He was driving a wagon load of "moonshine" down to town one day when the Revenue officers appeared on the scene. Tom left and left no trace. He doesn't even know what became of the "hoss" or the "licker." Last December the Captain gave Stewart a pass home. The railroad is 25 miles from his home and there was no way to go those 25 miles but to walk, so Stewart walked.

Stewart never puts his shoes on in the morning when he first wakes up. It makes no difference what time he gets up or how cold it is, Stewart goes around in his bare feet. Once he was asked why he did this he said, "The shoes are too cold and so are my feet. I wait until it gets warmer until I put my shoes on."

One time he was going to box Gregg. Well, Stewart squared off, wound up his arm and cringo!!!!

Gregg was a half an hour coming around.

March 4, 1918

Field hospital Number 33

The whole outfit left this morning for a two day hike. We took a complete field hospital with us which we borrowed from the 28th field hospital. The weather is rotten. Well we arrived at the camping grounds near Paw Creek N.C. and pitched the hospital. The boys did fairly well but they are a little rusty. Then they pitched their dog tents. It rained so hard and the ground is so sandy the dog tents would not stay "put" so everybody took

---

4. "French leave" is another way to say "A.W.O.L."

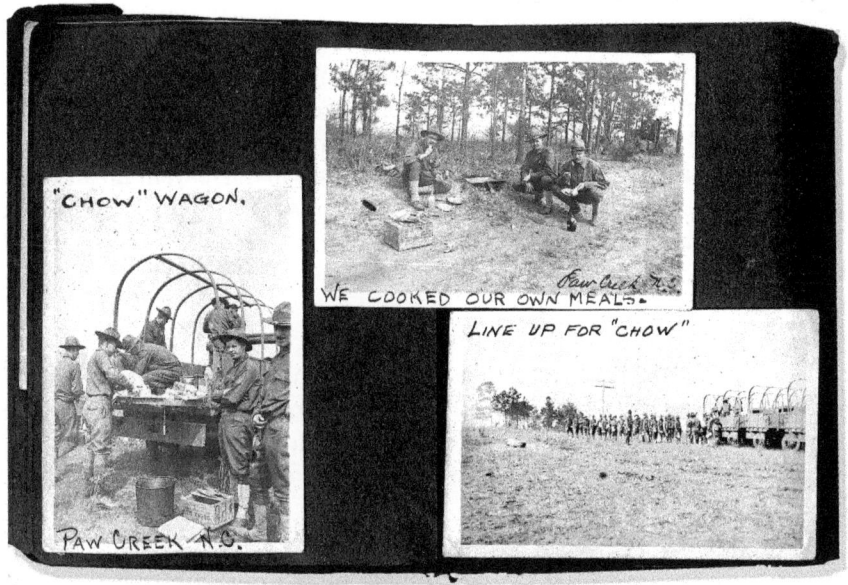

Field Hospital No. 33 on bivouac at Paw Creek, North Carolina (photo album).

shelter in the ward tents. The Victrola which was brought along was sure enjoyed.

Most of the boys were allowed to go to Paw Creek in the evening. It is some swell town—one road—one store and seven people. Great excitement prevailed in the town while the boys were their [sic] and the entire population turned out in masse to witness the event.

March 5

Still bad, misty weather this morning and Capt. Fitzpatrick gave the order to strike tents. This was done and they were put on the trucks and sent back to Camp Greene by 8:30 AM. The company then went out for a little ride. About 10 miles was covered and the sun came out and the outfit went for a walk through the woods. This was very much enjoyed. The big event was the walking across the creek on a fallen tree—Capt. Fitzpatrick waded out in the middle and acted as a life saver—he would have been recommended for a Carnegie Medal[5] for saving the life of Pvt. Thomas Burns but when private Carlin went across the log the captain didn't catch him and the result was that Carlin fell into water and took an unexpected bath.

---

5. The Carnegie Medal is a medallion awarded to civilians who risk their lives to an extraordinary degree saving or attempting to save the lives of others.

Felt sure that Carlin was going to die of shock because of the bath but thru the heroic efforts [of] Capt. Fitzpatrick and Lieutenants Slay and Herring, the man will probably survive. Back the company marched to the truck where we had mess and then had some practice bandaging wounded men. When we left this place on our homeward trip somebody saw something in the woods and called Sgt. Hodsdon's attention to it. He went up and Private Byam was sound asleep. After the excitement of getting Byam back on the truck had passed we beat it back to Camp Greene where all arrived safe, sound and tired.

March 6

Lieut. Dick and Private Wise went out on a motorcycle to meet the outfit yesterday and Wise succeeded in throwing a wheel and piling the Lieutenant up a six foot bank. That makes the fourth spill that the Lieutenant has had and Capt. Fitz swears that he will never ride in one of those things—

March 7

Pvt. Richard Zipse was discharged today—Poor Zipse he could not stand at attention. He would sway just like a tree in a wind storm—he received his diagnoses today. It was: "Constitutional psychopathic state Emotional Instability." Gee no wonder Zipse swayed. I guess I would too if I had to carry that around with me.

March 8, 1918

Sgt. Jongbloed and Pvt. John H. Page were transferred to the Hg. Field Hospital Section, Sanitary Train today. Sgt. Jongbloed is certainly a good man and his loss to the outfit is felt. Capt. Fitzpatrick stole him from Lieut. Turlington and now somebody comes along and swipes him from the Captain.

Supply officer of the Field Hospital Sec., Sanitary Train checked [picked] up all of the clothing today.

March 9, 1918

Inspection this morning was pretty bum. Pvt. Gorham, Barkman and Monahan placed under arrest for not having clean canteens at the inspection.

We got the Dodge car today—Now watch the fur fly—Hot Dog.

March 10, 1918

The Officers went out this afternoon to find a suitable camping grounds for the hike which the company is to take tomorrow. One private

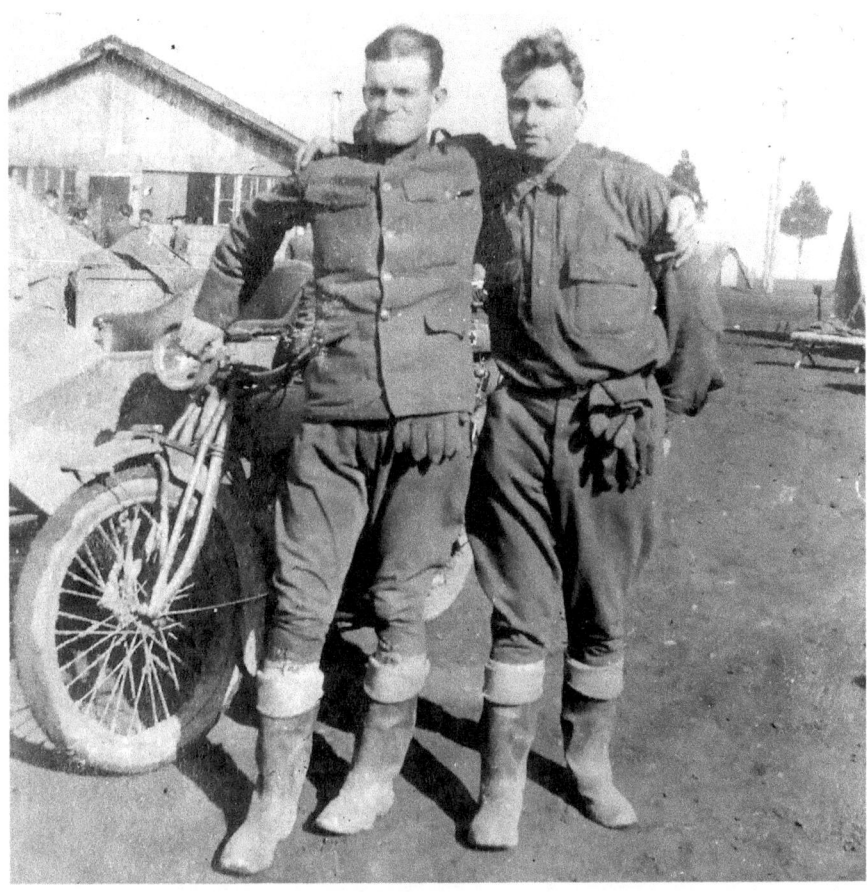

Privates Lawrence King and Edward Hind next to a sidecar-equipped Indian motorcycle at Camp Greene, North Carolina (photo album).

[was] assigned to Co. He is another drafted man. The boys are not giving any parties or dances for these conscripts. Things are pretty slow around here today. As Private DeWalt said, "Every day in the Army is like Sunday on the farm." DeWalt can't seem to find himself a girl for himself. He says that:—"Soldiers are about as popular as Ice Cream Soda at a Bar Tenders Picnic."

March 11, 1918

We are about 16 miles from Camp Greene and about 8 miles from Huntersville, N.C. We left Camp Greene about 8:30 and rode in the trucks 11 miles from Camp. Then the Company marched from there to where we are now. The name of this place, no one knows. It is just a place. On the way out we passed a schoolhouse. The school teacher invited us to come in. We did. She asked someone to say a few words and tell about the Soldiers. Sgt. Brown spoke for a minute or so and explained the medical beat to them. Then Pvt. Jordan sang "McCarthy's Party." This sure did bring down the house.[6]

March 12, 1918

Huntersville, N.C.

The outfit arrived here about 10:30 this morning and pitched camp. We are about a quarter of a mile from town. Small place but has quite a large school, two stories high with a large auditorium. Arrangements were made for a ball game and a basketball game. The baseball game was played.

Huntersville won 4–3. In the evening the outfit was invited to be the guests of the town. The people of Huntersville opened the school auditorium and the whole population turned out. The boys gave the show. Jordan, Arrowsmith and Lawrence sang and "Dodo" Lista did a "buck & wing"[7] while Private Barkman played a harmonica. After the Concert we

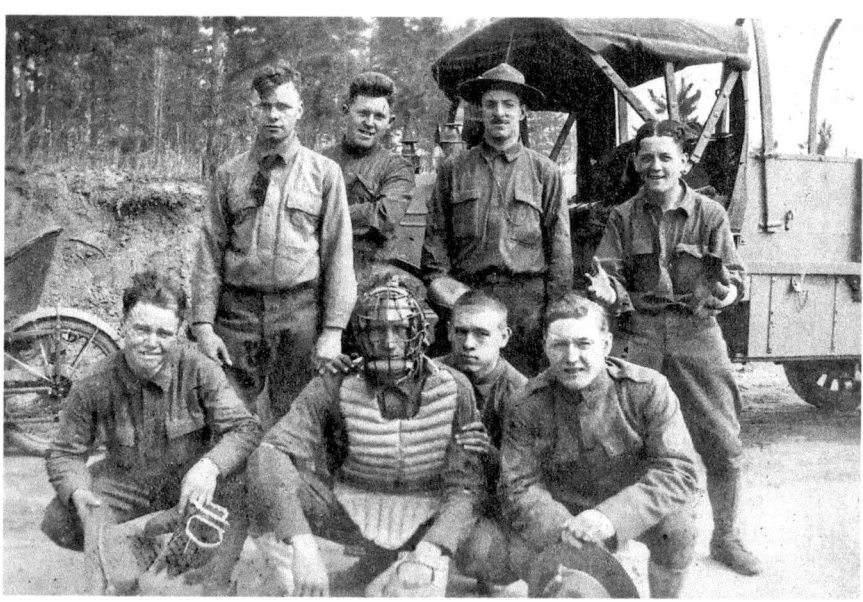

Field Hospital No. 33's "baseball team." Private Peter Lista is on the far right of the back row (photo album).

---

6. "McCarthy's Party" is an Irish drinking song.
7. "Buck & wing" is a tap dance step.

all went over to the "gym" and the Basket Ball game was played. Huntersville won this also. Score 32–16. After the game most of the fellas took a "chicken" home. I said "most" of the fellows took a chicken home; all did except Haney, Dewalt and Carlin. They didn't have chickens, they had little "peeps."[8]

March 13, 1918

Camp Greene, N.C.

Left Huntersville at 9:30 this morning and marched about 8 miles. Then ate mess and crawled into the trucks and rode back to Camp Greene. The boys are all tired but they sure are happy. They had the finest time they ever had in their army life and they are certainly do want to take another hike soon. The people of Huntersville treated them so nice that the men hated to leave.

March 14

Camp Greene, N.C.

A big wind storm all day. It didn't do any damage at all but it certainly did try awful hard—

Pvt. John Garden was released from Confinement. He says, "Never again."

March 15, 1918

Camp Greene, N.C.

Pvt. Frederick A Spang sent to base hospital. He is going to have his belly opened—Pvt. Frank D. Barkman is going to be discharged—T.B.

March 16, 1918

Camp Greene

The Inspection this morning was fine. The Captain said that it was the best ever. Major Wilmerding inspected all Sanitary Formations in the Fourth Division and couldn't find a fault in anything.

Mrs. Fitzpatrick was to come to Charlotte yesterday but their train was late. She expects to arrive tomorrow morning at 6:35.

Private Sadowski is a hot sketch. He can't understand English. Lieut.

---

8. The *Charlotte Observer* reported of the Field Hospital No. 33 encounter with the people of Hunersville: "...the soldiers gave a most enjoyable impromptu concert, and many of those present availed themselves of the opportunity of meeting the khaki-clad boys. Patriotic songs were sung, and altogether it was an evening of great pleasure. The soldiers, by their courtesy and gentlemanly bearing, won not only the goodwill, but the respect of the people." The article did note the games they played, but there was no mention of any "chickens" or "peeps."

Dick asked him what he was doing with the manure. He told the lieutenant that he was feeding it to the mules.

Yesterday Lieut. Dick was out in the motorcycle. Lieut. Dick asked Carlin if he had _____ lately. Carlin said "_____ have been _____." Lieut. Dick said, "What did you think" I said. "You _____ did _____ any _____."

Carlin is wondering lately yet why the lieutenant laughed. Today is Alan's birthday.[9]

Sunday, Mar 17

Camp Greene, N.C.
Not much doing today. Getting ready for a three day hike.

Monday, March 18, 1918

Newell N.C.

Private Rizzo took the Dodge into Charlotte to get the Captain to bring him back to camp. On his way to town he wrapped it around the end of a freight car. The Captain did not complement him any on the job but took a second look at the car and fired him.

MOTTO:—Never attempt to do exterior decorating on a freight car with a Dodge Automobile.

With the exception of the above episode we succeeded leaving Camp Greene and reaching the outskirts of the city of Charlotte. Then we hiked for four miles and had mess. After mess we piled in the trucks and rode to Newell, N.C. We pitched camp and here we are. Lots of visitors in camp. There are not many "chickens" in this town. It's so slow that it makes me sleepy.

March 19, 1918

Rocky River, N.C.

Broke camp and marched six miles and then rode to this place in the trucks. There's not even a town near here. Captain has requested Sgt. Hoyt to get permission from Maj. Wilmerding for us to stay out for a few days longer. It looks like rain and I suppose we are in for some bad weather.

March 20, 1918

Near Concord, N.C.

We are about a mile from Concord. The roads are so bad that the trucks can't go any farther. I said "we" but the truth is that the only people

---

9. Alan Benson Brown, Leland's brother, was born on March 16, 1903, and died on December 15, 1978.

in camp are Sgt. Brown; he is in charge of quarters and Sergeant of the Guard; Private Eberly and he is sick; and Private Borowsky and he is under arrest. The rest of the whole outfit is in Concord. We left Rocky River and came here. Then the trucks got stuck. Carlin and Sergeant Brown were in one of the motorcycles and it broke down. Carlin stayed with the machine and the Sergeant came to camp. The truck picked up Carlin and left Borowsky on guard. When the truck came back to where the motorcycle was, Borowsky had disappeared. He was found about a quarter mile away taking it easy on a rail fence. He was put under arrest for being off post. Carlin was to bring another motorcycle out from Camp Greene. He came into Camp about 11 PM. His cycle was stalled about 4 miles from here—

March 21, 1918

Rocky River (Again)
Ate mess here and left for Newell, N.C. where we are to stay tonight.
Newell, N.C.
Boys hiked here from Rocky River all dead tired. The people here opened the schoolhouse and we gave them an entertainment. We sure had one grand time. I wish we did not have to go in tomorrow.

March 22, 1918

Camp Greene, N.C.
Arrived back to Camp Greene at noon in time for mess. The medical property for the hospital arrived today and is all packed in the supply tent. Most everybody [is] tired and in bed asleep at 9 P.M.

March 23 Camp Greene

Inspection this morning. Fairly good. We expect to go on another hike next week.

March 24, Sunday

A mean cold rainy day—Six of the men who were out on special duty at the Base Hospital came back to duty with the company—Eight Privates who were drafted were assigned to us for rations.
One of Lieut. Dick's Lady Friends arrived in camp this afternoon. Does not look much as if we were going to take the hike tomorrow. The weather is rotten.
News came today that a big battle was being fought around St. Quentin. The information says that things are going bad for the English. The attack is costing lots of German lives. It will be a costly victory for

Germany.[10] Germany apparently has a gun which throws a 9½ inch projectile 62 miles. It hardly seems possible that such is the truth. Maj. Gen. Cameron[11] issued a statement in which he says that he believes it to be true, but that the United States has a war machine which will go the Germans one better. I knew that we would have the jump on them and we are going to keep it too.[12]

March 25, 1918

We did not go this morning. Probably leave tomorrow. New[s] received this morning confirmed the fact that the British are slowly retreating. Unofficial information states that the British have captured three Army divisions of Germans. 80,000 men-some bunch.

March 26, 1918

Left Camp Greene, N.C.
Arrived 2 miles from Pineville N.C. Went to town. Some dead place.

March 27, 1918

Pineville, N.C.
Usual hike duties. The town had us give our usual concert. Then the ladies of the town who were dressed as Red Cross nurses served us punch and cake. Some treat.

March 28, 1918

Marched 5 miles from Pineville and then rode back to the town. The people had baked biscuits and sent some sandwiches down to the men.

---

10. The battle that he mentions near Saint-Quentin was the result of a big push by the Germans hoping that a quick advance near Paris would bring the Allies to the bargaining table before a large number of American troops could arrive in France, tipping the balance against them. The Germans were realizing that they were reaching the breaking point and needed a decisive victory. Although they did advance, it was less than they had wished.

11. Major General George H. Cameron was the first commander of the Army's 4th Division and led it from its first organization at Camp Greene, North Carolina, through most of 1918. In August of that year, he commanded the V Corps. His performance during the battle of Montfaucon led to conflict with the First United States Army's chief of staff, Hugh Drum, which resulted in his relief from that command. He was also thought to be responsible for designing the 4th Division's shoulder patch.

12. The large gun that Sergeant Brown referred to is the German Army's "Paris Gun." It was capable of firing eight- to nine-inch shells up to 80 miles. Although impractical as an ordinary artillery weapon due to its inaccuracy, it was thought that it was used as a weapon of terror in France and, more specifically, Paris. It was built by the Krupp factory and could only be fired 50 to 60 times before it had to be rebored due to the tremendous wear of the high-velocity shells on the barrel of the gun.

Chapter 1. Camp Greene

March 29, 1918

Arrived at Camp Greene at 10 this morning. Everybody cleaning up for inspection.

March 30, 1918

No inspection. The outfit moved all of their motor trucks over to where the 47th seventh infantry used to be. We are all going to Gastonia N.C. to the Artillery Range to be the Camp Hospital.

April 1, 1918

Whole outfit moved to Camp Chronicle today and took over the hospital.[13] Busy getting things straightened out. Everything is in working order. There is a bad case of acute appendicitis here. The chap is likely to die.

April 2, 1918

Five cases received today. Three slightly injured. One a little fella seven years old [was] struck by shrapnel. He is in bad shape. The other fellow was struck and run over by some horses. The appendicitis case died this morning. The Dodge with the Captain, Pvt. Zollers and some Colonel were fired at by a Battery. They sure did duck.

April 3

Camp Chronicle
Pvt. Frank Waenberghe went home today to Mishawaka, Wisconsin.[14]

April 4

Sgt. Leland N. Brown appointed Sergeant First Class, Medical Department to rank from April 3, 1918.

April 5, 1918

Nothing new strange or startling. Only joy in life seems to be playing "Old Maid" except for the times when we take swimming lessons in the stew trying to locate a piece of 1898 Model Beef but we like it.

---

13. Camp Chronicle was at or near Gastonia, North Carolina, which is about 10 miles west of Charlotte, North Carolina.
14. This is the only reference to Private Frank Waenberghe in the diary. He shipped and returned to the United States with Field Hospital No. 33. He was a shoemaker, born in Belgium in 1898, and became a U.S. citizen after he served in 1919. Source: 1920 U.S. Census, Mishawaka, Indiana, and the U.S. Army Transport Service Passengers Lists

April 6, 1918

Still at Camp Chronicle with the hospital inspection this morning. Just a hasty glance through the tents. Nothing except a flock of flying oysters flew over today.[15] Went so fast we did not have a chance to kill any. Private Lawrence wants to have his voice cultivated so he came to the surgeons about it. They recommended that he have his throat cut. Everybody agreed.

April 7, 1918

Sunday. Camp Chronicle, N. C.
Not a new case today.
Everything [is] slow as the deuce. Lollypop entertained the patients by playing the violin. The Signal Corps across the hollow enjoyed it so much they are tearing down the brick building and are going to present to him on the installment plan.

April 8, 1918

Blue Monday and it is blue. Rained all night and all day. How the hell can anyone expect anything to happen when things go like this?

April 18, 1918

Camp Chronicle
Still on the job as Camp Hospital. Capt. Fitzpatrick, Lt. Johnson and Lt. Dick left Camp Greene today for Europe. Lieutenant Slay is in command of the outfit.

April 19, 1918

This camp is to be abandoned next Tuesday.

April 22, 1918

Packed up on the 20th and 21st. Some of the men came back to Camp Greene. The balance arrived today. We are located in new quarters. They are much nicer than the old ones.
It's as hot as the deuce.

April 23, 1918

Camp Greene, N.C
We are beginning to pack up for overseas duty. The outfit is doing fatigue work as usual.

---

15. The assumption is that there were some oysters available but only a few and that they were gone before he had a chance to have any.

Chapter 1. Camp Greene

April 30, 1918

Had a banquet last night. It sure was a success. All commanding officers of the Sanitary Train are present. Everybody in the outfit has a menu so there is no use in trying to tell much about it.

May 1–7

Usual Camp duties. The outfit is packing the stuff for over-seas duty. Pvt. Shearer returned from the guard-house. Private Sutton[16] was sentenced to one month confinement at hard labor. His sentence began April 25, 1918. We are to take him with us. Privates Walter Wigington and Philip Enwright [are] A.W.O.L.

Tuesday, May 7, 1918

Word was received that private Shearer was A.W.O.L. again.

May 8, 1918

Orders were received to have our stuff all packed on a train by 10 o'clock tomorrow morning. It looks as if we are off to Europe at last. The boys are working like slaves. They are going to be on the job all night and they have to pack all the automobiles for the whole Sanitary Train.

May 9

Everything packed. Left for Philadelphia to attend my grandmother's funeral.[17]

Monday, May 13, 1918

I arrived back in Camp Greene at 8 AM too tired to eat. At 10 o'clock I went to the R.R. station and at 2 o'clock the train pulled out for PORT OF EMBARKATION.

Oh, Boy, oh Joy where do we go from here. We are off on a wonderful experience at last. I at last admit that we are going to Europe. It seems too good to be true. We are balling the jack for the north. Just passed Danville, Va. Think I will turn in.

Sgt. First Class Hodsdon and Sgt. First Class Steven S. Lombard are sharing the compartment with me.

---

16. Private Sutton was the soldier who was caught malingering.
17. His grandmother was his father's mother: Annie Elizabeth Nelson Brown, November 28, 1841–May 9, 1918.

May 14, 1918, Tuesday

Camp Merritt, N.J.[18]

Awoke this morning in Washington, D.C. Passed through Baltimore, Philadelphia, Trenton and Jersey City then up to Camp Merritt. This is a swell place. We have barracks and spring beds with mattresses. Some class.

Wednesday, May 15, 1918

Made out the passenger lists today. Some job. There is nothing to do but await transportation across now.

Thursday, May 16, 1918

Camp Merritt

Field hospitals #19 and #21 and ambulance companies #19 and #21 from Fort Riley, Kansas, arrived yesterday.

Friday Phila. Pa, May 17, 1918

Ambulance companies #28 and #33 sailed for Europe today. I was given a pass and went home to Philadelphia. Saw a great many people I knew.[19]

Saturday, Camp Merritt, May 18, 1918

Arrived back at camp at 9 a.m. and slept all day.

Sunday, Phila, Pa., May 19, 1918

Beat it to Philadelphia again this morning and Marian and I went to church today.

Monday, May 20, 1918

Camp Merritt, New Jersey
Back again, Slept all day.

May 21, 1918

Philadelphia, Pa.

Sgt. Hodsdon and Dewalt and I went to Phila. this morning. Went to Keith's tonight.[20]

---

18. Camp Merritt, New Jersey, is northwest of Tenafly on the west side of the Hudson River and about 10 miles from New York City.

19. Hospital Companies 19, 21, 28, and 33, as well as Ambulance Companies 28 and 33, were all attached to the 4th Division.

20. Keith's Chestnut Street Theatre was mostly a theater for vaudeville acts.

Chapter 1. Camp Greene

Wednesday, May 22, 1918

Camp Merritt, New Jersey
We stayed in Collingdale[21] overnight and came back to camp this morning. Slept all afternoon.

Thursday, May 23, 1918

Camp Merritt N.J.
Guess we are going to leave here Sunday. Weighed all of our baggage and expect to be ready to take the boat at 8 A.M. Sunday.

May 24, 1918

Friday, Camp Merritt, N.J.
Worked in the morning. I went over to New York in the afternoon. Had a swell time. Went to see aunt Annie Brown.[22] She took me out to dinner and then we walked over to Riverside Drive and took a 5th Avenue bus downtown. Saw Schwabs, Gould, Vanderbilt residences. Had to come back by 11 o'clock. Everything [is] fine. There is to be a physical inspection at 10 o'clock tomorrow.

Saturday, May 25, 1918

Packed our barrack bag & carried them to the station. I passed the Physical Examination.

---

21. Sergeant Brown was living with his parents in Collingdale before he enlisted. Collingdale is about 10 miles southwest of Philadelphia.
22. Annie Brown was the wife of his uncle Herbert Brown.

Chapter 2

AT SEA

Sunday May 26, 1918

R.M.S. "Melita"[1]

Got up at 3:30 AM left Camp Merritt at 5:30 A.M. and marched to Creshill [Cresskill] and took the Erie R.R. to Jersey City. Then the ferry across to New York and then up the gangplank on board the Royal Mail Steamship Melita. The company is assigned quarters in the steerage. Sgt. Hodsdon, Lombard and I are in the first cabin forward on the starboard side. Hodsdon and I are together. We have a peach of a place. The men line up with mess kits for chow. We eat a real dinner with real china and silverware—It sure is great.

Monday, May 27, 1918

We left New York in a fog at 7 A.M. Passed the statue while we were eating breakfast. Learned that we have quite an important person on board. Premier Borden of Canada. The seas are quite smooth and very few are sick.

Tuesday, May 28, 1918

R.M.S. "Melita"
Second day out

The sea still continues smooth. We left New York yesterday morning there was quite a fog. This has continued more or less all the time since. The foghorns blew all night long. I sure am hungry and eat everything that comes on the table. The ship is in the center of the entire bunch in the convoy. It is carrying the Premier of Australia and New Zealand beside the Canadian. It also has a bunch of silver in the hold. It will be the best taken care of ship in the whole bunch.

---

1. Th was built for the Canadian Pacific Railroad in Glasgow, Scotland, in 1918. She was 425 feet in length and 67 feet in breadth. The *Melita* survived German U-boats transporting troops from North America to Europe during World War I but met her fate in 1941 when she sank after being bombed at Tobruk Roads, Libya.

Chapter 2. At Sea

I was quite surprised that the color of the water. When you look down it seems to be black.

There is life belt drill twice a day. A Regular Army Major is in charge of it. He spoke about it like this: "When you men come out on deck you are not to smoke or talk. You are to stand at attention and not to do anything until you were told. In case of emergency you are to find your place on deck and await further orders. This is essential for your safety. Any officer finding any man disobeying the smallest order [he] will instantly shoot him. I will back him up on it."

These were some orders but discipline is certainly essential to safety in case we are torpedoed.

Tobacco was distributed today. Each enlisted man received one package of cigarettes, one can of Velvet Tobacco, one package of Cigarette Papers and one plug of Star Chewing Tobacco.

The life belt drill is worked like this. The bugler blows the call to quarters. Every man goes to quarters and puts on his life belt. Then first call is sounded and immediately. "Assembly." It takes about six minutes for the men to get out on deck. Then the First Sergeant calls the role and the bunch are dismissed.

At night all the port-holes are fastened and bolted and curtains are hung on the inside as a double precaution. I just looked out of my port-hole (5:45 P.M.) and there is the cruiser which has been with us ever since we left New York. She keeps right opposite us all the time. The fog has kept her hidden and this is the first time I have seen her today. There's one thing I am glad of [that] she is an American. We passed her in New York Harbor. That is how I know her nationality. I saw some of Uncle Sam's Jackies and Marines on her.[2]

May 29, 1918

R.M.S. "Melita"
Third Day Out

Pretty rough. The waves are breaking over the forward deck and there is a good many men sick. I am not sick but I am next thing to it. Our cruiser has left us. Suppose she is on the other side of the convoy. Had life belt drill this morning and are going to have it again this afternoon.

June 1, 1918

R.M.S. "Melita"
Sixth Day Out Saturday

---

2. "Jackies" are American sailors.

Finished the payroll today. This last week sure has been a busy one for me. One week ago today I was talking [taking?] dinner with Aunt Annie and now I am in the middle of the Atlantic. Day before yesterday was one rough day. I was seasick. The sea ran so high that it washed over our decks. It was Memorial Day and I wonder how the folks at home are enjoying themselves. They must know by now that I have left. Yesterday the rough weather had gone and I felt much better.

American money was exchanged for English yesterday. We had to take the fellas word for what we got. One did not know the difference. I have 60 cents worth of it. Only have a quarter and a dime in the United States money left. I am going to keep them for pocket pieces.

Today is as fine and clear a day as anyone would want. This boat has two 6 inch depth bomb mortars and one 6" gun. There was gun practice this afternoon. The cruiser put a flag out for us to shoot at. The mortar refused to work so they used the 6" gun. Boy oh Boy but she sure did make a racket when she went off. Two shots to get the range. The third hit the flag and so did the fourth. I think that we can trust those gunners. They are English sailors.

June 2, 1918

R.M.S. "Melita"
Sunday Seventh Day out.
Sea became rough this afternoon again. It has been raining since noon. Life belt drill at 10:30 and 2 today. Church services this morning and this afternoon. I found out about some of the ships in the fleet. There are 13 merchantmen. The battleship which is convoying us is the New Hampshire. Among the merchantmen is one which is a converted cruiser. Another of the ships is carrying munitions. Another is the "Celtic." Two others belong to the new class which are being built by the British Government. They are known as Standard Ships. They are named after leaves. These two happen to be the "Silver Leaf" and the "Rose Leaf."

I stopped smoking last night.

June 3, 1918

R.M.S. "Melita"
Monday. Eighth Day Out
Hodsdon is sitting in his birth. He says he is well for the first time in eight days. He is a good soldier but he can't brag about the sailor. Rained most of the day. Had life belt drill as usual. It is getting cold and it is getting colder every minute. Our course seems to be a little northeast of North. Goodness knows where we are heading for. I spent some of my English money today. Gave the fellow a shilling. He gave me seven coins

back. Goodness knows how much they are worth. Went over the company fund today. We are $13.15 short. Lieut. Herring is just raising the roof.

Saw several schools of fish swimming near the surface. Saw a small whale spouting about a quarter a mile from the ship. The eats are still good. Started to smoke again today.

Letter to family, "At Sea" May 1918

This is the first letter to you since I sailed and left the U.S.A. Let me tell you about the swell accommodations which I have. I share a state room on a large liner with Sgt. Hodsdon. He has the upper, I the lower birth. We are on the starboard side and have a state room right on the outside and therefore have a porthole. We also have a private wash stand in our room. Electric lights and service of the steward all the time. Put our shoes out at night and they are polished in the morning. We have our meals served in the main dining room salon. The same place that the officers eat except that we eat a half hour before they do. The meals are served in courses and they are well cooked. No Army chow but real food. We have a printed menu and it sure is great.

I wish I could tell you about the ship itself but that is not permitted. My goodness but will I not have a bunch of stuff to tell you about when I see you again.

June 4, 1918

Ninth Day Out
R.M.S. "Melita" Tuesday

Went to an entertainment last night. It was held in the main dining room. The talent was furnished by members of the A.E.F. onboard.[3] Premier Borden was chairman of the evening. We had a good time. Entertainment was for the benefit of the Disabled Marines. A collection was taken and the proceeds amounted to about $165.00.

Sunday, June 9, 1918

Winchester England

Well diary, at last we have set our foot on foreign soil. Friday morning they tumbled us out of bed at 3:30 and we were just entering the North Channel and passing between Ireland and Scotland. This was the most dangerous part of the whole voyage. I forgot to say that on Wednesday morning we woke to find ourselves surrounded by English Destroyers, those greyhounds of the sea. They are little boats and they sit low in the water. They sure do remind me of a greyhound. They are continually circling around the boat. They followed us clear into port. Soon after we

---

3. The AEF was the American Expeditionary Forces under the command of General John J. Pershing.

entered the North Channel a dirigible picked us up and then another. It stayed with us until we entered the mouth of the Mercy River. This is a big, dirty river with a very strong current. We passed the Isle of Man in the Irish Sea. England has a big German detention camp here. We laid all night in Liverpool harbor. The people cheered us all the way up the river. We passed Brighton Beach and Blackpool [which] are two English seaside resorts. I stayed up all night. We started to unload and did not finish and get off the boat until about 10 o'clock.

At the wharf we were met by a mounted policeman. He resembled a clown more than a policeman. He had a hat on his head which made him look like Happy Hooligan. Well he escorted us to the train sheds. I saw my first English train. The coaches are divided into compartments. There is first, second and third class.

Each compartment holds eight men. Well we passed through Sheffield, Banbury Cross and I saw Oxford. The university buildings are beautiful. England is a beautiful country. It is rolling and hilly and reminds me of a gigantic garden. It is beyond me in description. There is no place in the coaches to urinate so the boys just relieve themselves out the window. You could look out and see half a dozen streams going at once. Red Cross fed us twice. The people have not cheered us as the people in the United States do. Some years of war have about taken the pep out of them. They simply applaud. There were very few men and most of the women were in black. There was one old lady looking at us and if ever pity was written in one's eyes, it was in hers.

We arrived at Winchester last night and marched 4 miles to the camp which is on Lord Derby's place on the Salisbury Plains. It is an English camp and we hardly get enough to eat. This British ration is rotten. We are resting up today and are going to cross to France tomorrow.

Letter to family, June 9, 1918

Of course you have received my safe arrival card by this time. The trip was all I expected and I enjoyed every minute of it. I had fine quarters with Sergeant Hodsdon. We only had one day where the weather was anyway rough. I was seasick then but I soon got used to the motion and I felt no inconvenience after that. Before we landed the land that we saw was certainly beautiful. The towns that we passed thru are beyond description as far as I can do. The country that we passed thru is the best ordered that I have ever seen in my life. I do not mean by this that you see prettier scenery than in the U.S. but the approaches which you find when you enter a city are simply great. You know that the American Railroads as a rule run into the worst part of a town and there are always railroad yards but there is not true of the towns I have passed thru. You see mile after mile of rolling land under cultivation. There are no woods and high trees.

Chapter 2. At Sea

We have reached our camp. I suppose from now on we will be more or less on the move all the time. I hope so, for I sure have become a gypsy. I hate to be in the same place very long.

I had my hair cut today. Sgt. Bowman cut mine and I cut his. You can imagine how we looked when we got thru with each other. I want to hear all the news about Philly and all there is about Darby.

Tell me all you can about the war. I have not heard a bit of war news for three weeks. The papers here seem to avoid it. They limit everything to just official reports. The papers here are the funniest thing you ever saw. The Smyrna Times is a big city journal beside the things that they sell and call newspapers. Four pages, about four columns of news and all the rest is ads.

Chapter 3

FRANCE

Wednesday, June 12, 1918

Le Havre, France

We left Winchester, England, and proceeded to Southampton, England, by rail. We were loaded onto transport and left England at dusk for France. I slept on the deck and had some life preservers for pillows. I had a good night's sleep except that it was cold. There were a lot of English soldiers on the boat. They have been wounded and recovered and were being shipped back to the front. There were some English recruits on board too. They were scared stiff. The wounded men were typical of all English soldiers I have met. They are yellow cowards. All they think is how soon they will get wounded again so they can get out of it. I heard dozens of them saying that they had shot themselves so they could be sent back to England. One soldier said he had shot himself in the hand last time and this time he is going to shoot himself in the leg. It looks to me as if France and United States will have to do this scrapping themselves.

We arrived Le Havre, France, and then marched to an English Rest Camp on the outskirts of the town. The barracks of the men are nothing but stable stalls. The grub is furnished by the English. It consists mostly of cheese and bread and tea. Does not suit a Yankee at all. In the afternoon we were marched up on a hill overlooking the town and we were issued a gas mask. And we were put through the gas chamber to test the mask. Mine was all right.

Letter to family, June 12, 1918

> *Now I can talk some more and a little more freely than I have been able to. To begin with I am "Somewhere in France" and just as happy as if I were back in Georgia or Carolina. Of course not quite as well satisfied as if I were in Collingdale but I am not homesick. ...you know how much I wanted to cross the ocean but I always felt scared about it. There was not a minute's worry on the whole trip. I liked it so much that I almost wish that I had enlisted in the Navy instead of the Army.*

Chapter 3. France

People in the states cheered us as we went along but the people over here have gotten past that point. They applaud or run out to take a hold of your hand just to touch you. They think a great lot of the Americans. Then we passed through the town from the ship to the railroad. We marched in a column through the main street.

The procession was headed by a Mounted policeman. I can't describe him. He was beyond description. I supposed he looked real enough to the civilians who have seen him all their life, but not to me. If the City Troop of Phila. would put on a bell boy hat and black trous[ers], he would be the policeman.

I saw one woman who was watching us as we marched by and if there was pity written on anyone's face it was on hers. Well we called to her and joshed her and she soon brightened up. She said her son had been in it for two and a half years and she always thought of him when she saw troops marching along. We took a tram to our camp and passed some of he prettiest cities and towns in England. People came to the tram to feed us and give us newspapers. Those papers were the first we have seen for almost two weeks and we had almost forgotten that things were happening in the world. The British red cross met us at several stations and gave us food and cigarettes.

Then we arrived at our rest camp. I saw some mighty pretty country and some beautiful estates. I saw some castles too. They are magnificent to look at. Well we left the rest camp and proceeded to the port from which we embarked for France. The trip across the channel was some trip. That is all. Now I am in France. It reminds me very much of the U.S. I mean the layout of the country.

I haven't had a bath for two weeks but I am promised one tomorrow morning. The reason for this is that we have been on the move almost all the time. The letters I have written over here are the hardest I have ever written because there is so much to tell and I can't say a word about it. I'll close now and beat it to bed. It is 7:30 PM now 1:30 AM in Philadelphia. I am going to bed while you in Philadelphia are in the middle of the day.

The days here are the longest I have ever seen. It is light until 11, then it starts to get light again about 2:30 in the morning. The nights are cold and days are very hot. Tell Alan that the cars are marked Hommes 40 Chevaux 20 just as he said they would be.[1]

Saturday morning, June 15, 1918.

Meaux, France

We stayed at the rest camp at Le Havre. I went into Le Havre to see the town. There were two things which impress themselves on my American mind. The first was the harlots which are in the city in great numbers. Their ages run from 16 to 60. You will be walking on the street and a swell looking dame will come up to you and say good evening and without further words hand you her license for her trade and then show you her health certificate showing she has no venereal disease. I guess we have plenty of them in the states but none are as open about it as they are here.

The second thing which I noticed was an elderly man walk out of a

---

1. As the letters home were transcribed by his parents, they may have miswritten that the railroad cars are labeled 20 chevaux instead of 10.

wine shop and back up against the wall and urinate. Women were passing but they paid no attention to him or he to them. I saw a girl about 20 years old go to the curb and squat and relieve herself. By George but this sure is some funny country and they call themselves civilized.

Well we left there and marched to the station at Le Havre. We rode in freight cars which bore the sign (Hommes 40 Chevaux 8–10) which means men 40, Horses 8 to 10. In other words I was to travel in a cattle car. Some class. Everything went along O.K. until night. There was only 31 men in my car and by laying all over each other is possible for just 30 of us find a room to lay down to sleep.

I got out and went up and slept on the roof of the car. It was dangerous but it was the best place to sleep. When we woke up in the morning we were 3 miles from Paris. We did not pass thru but around it. I saw the Eiffel Tower and the big cathedral. Our train pulled up beside a train load of French soldiers. We sure had a good time with them. I met a young fellow and we talked for a long time.[2] The train pulled out and took us to Meaux. This is the nearest point which the Germans were to Paris in fall of 1914. The town has been bombed and shows signs of it. It is close to the fighting line now. We have met the rest of the Division and here we are.

Saturday night, June 15, 1918

Pierre Levee, France

We have been moved. We marched to this place today. We are at a farm house close to the lines. Once in a while the guns can be heard. I am sleeping in a manger. Is the best bed that I have had since I got off the boat. The straw is clean and it is free from lice.

Sunday, June 16 1918

Pierre Levee, France

Sure was some fighting last night. The German Aeroplane tried to cross our lines. The searchlight picked it up and finally brought it down. It fell [in] a mess of flames.

I have been busy today making out reports. We are in immediate reserve behind the lines. The commanding general says we are to move in a minutes notice. The Chaplain held services in the courtyard. I attended.

Monday, June 17, 1918

Pierre Levee, France

Captain Fitzpatrick and Lieut. Johnson came to report for duty. I certainly was glad to see them.

---

2. The young fellow he mentions here was probably Jean Cherfils, who sent him a postcard in August 1918. That postcard is shown and transcribed in the appendix.

Received news that the Germans had driven our forces back across the Marne. We ordered a new Field Hospital today. We had horse meat for breakfast. It has a strong taste that I did not like.

Tuesday, June 18, 1918

Pierre Levee, France

There was an aeroplane battle almost overhead this morning but the German succeeded in getting away. We had gas mask drill today. I wore mine for 50 minutes this morning and 45 minutes [in the] afternoon. I'll tell you it sure is torture. Lieutenant Dick came in today. These men have been all over the American lines.

Friday, June 21, 1918

Pierre Levee, France

We moved to another part of the town yesterday. We are occupying a Chateau near the firing line.[3] It is some swell place. We are going to open a hospital here.

Letter to family, June 21, 1918

I have been in Europe two weeks today but I have had no mail from home. We are in service now. Doing real work on the line. We are occupying an old French estate. I hope I can describe it to you. The house or castle or Chateau is built in the form of a U.

The entire grounds are surrounded by a wall about 6 feet high running in the direction as spokes in a wheel, with the house as the hub, are wide lanes or walks. Trees are planted along the sides of these walks. These trees are trimmed so that the branches on the inside do not begin to try to meet the branches from the other side until about 50 feet from the ground. The result of this is a high natural, arched walk exactly as I have seen in paintings but which I always believe that existed only in the brain of an artist. The rich French seem to delight in the cultivation of forests where every tree was in line with the tree next to it—and believe me the lines sure were straight.

Coming back to the house the first thing you see is the moat. You cross it and enter a room. The floor is inlaid hardwood. The ceiling is 15 feet high and there are 5 large mirrors in the room. These run from floor to ceiling. Windows, which are many, also run from floor to ceiling. The space between the windows is paneled off. No wallpaper here, instead you find leather. The family coat of arms is on the leather. Two other rooms, one on each side of this room, are furnished about the same except that curtains cover the walls. The walls separating these rooms can be pushed back and the whole thrown into one room. There are about nine smaller rooms on the first floor. They contain nothing of special interest except for the many ways of getting in and out of them. The second floor contains the bedrooms. The beds are set in the wall and have canopies over them. The third floor contains more bedrooms but these were probably used by servants.

Most of the furniture has been moved but what is left is certainly a delight to me.

---

3. Château de Montebise

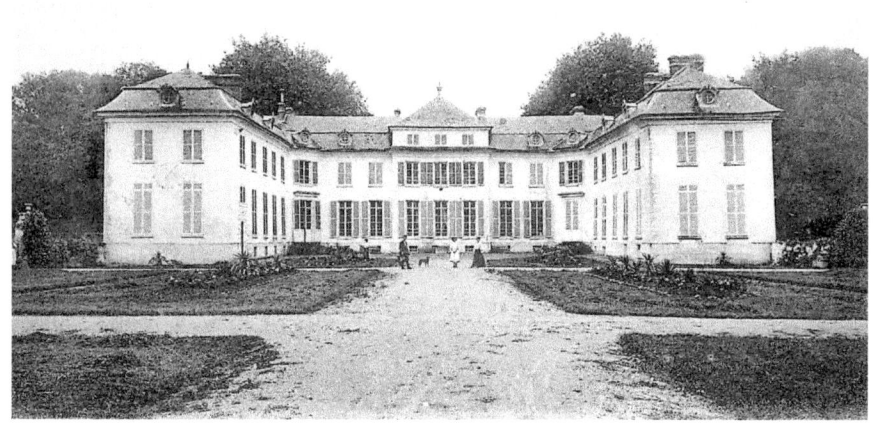

An early 20th-century postcard showing Château de Montebise, where Sergeant Brown was quartered (Will Brown Collection).

The cellar contains the kitchen and the dungeons. The dungeon is an interesting place but I would rather live on the outside. I have a room on the top floor. I can go to my window and see the American trenches, the German trenches and "no man's land." The guns go all the time. Aeroplanes are in the air all the time and every once in a while you can see an air battle. Today I got a German gas mask but it is too big to lug around with me.

I am well and I am enjoying it just the same as I have enjoyed every minute I have been in the Army.

Capt. Fitzpatrick, Lieut. Johnson and Lieut. Dick are with us again. We are going to be paid Monday. Before the war a French franc was worth 20¢. Now we get five francs and 71 centimes for every dollar.

Sunday, June 23, 1918

Pierre Levee, France

We received our first patients last night. The place was one busy place then. The men are just sick. None have been fighting as yet. The Fourth Division is still in reserve in the defense of Paris.

The women of New Zealand have formed a society similar to the Y.W.C.A. It is to look out for their soldiers in France. They secured services for first class clean whores in France and they are for use of the New Zealand troops only. This place is in Paris.

Chapter 3. France

June 25, 1918

The outfit was paid off yesterday. We are still receiving and shipping patients. There was an American officer sent in from the line today. He had a piece of paper and a tale. He was standing in the front line trench and a large high explosive came over and struck just behind them but did not explode. They, he and a few other officers, went over and unscrewed the cap to make it safe and just under the cap was a piece of paper. This was open[ed] and it read "A Tommy has done his last bit."

Our boys captured a kilometer of trenches last night and this morning they had consolidated them with ours.

Letter to family, June 25, 1918

One month ago today I left the US. We are still at the Chateau. I have seen all there is to see at this place and want to move on again. This is how I have always felt when I have been stationed at a place very long. Yesterday was payday. I received our pay for the month of May. I just finished the payroll for the month of June and I suppose we will be paid again in about a week or 10 days. We are paid in French money. It is not hard to learn. I think I have gotten it straight. In times of peace our dollar was worth only 5 Francs. But now our dollar is worth 5 francs and 70 centimes and the government gives us the benefit of this and does not charge us any exchange on the money. You see that I made about 17 francs on my American money when I was paid. I paid all my debts and bought some tobacco, cakes and chewing gum and some candy. There is little chance for me to spend money.

One of the officers went into a large town near here today and bought a bunch of tobacco and etc., and he sold out in about a half an hour. Tooth paste been hard to get. I have been trying to buy some ever since we came to France, but the stores do not seem to keep it. I do not think the people take as much care of their teeth as we do in the U.S.

Soap is another scarce article. I have about four pounds of it with me. No one sells it. It was pretty heavy at times and I have wanted to throw it away but I still have it and am thankful for it.

It is really true that we hear less about the war than you do the States. Our news is limited to the official statements. There are no articles such as you find in American papers. We get the news of the world in the Paris edition of the New York Herald and Chicago Tribune. We get the papers early in the morning. They cost us 15 centimes. That is three cents.

Last night Sgt. Hodsdon and I bought a fresh cheese. The farmers about this part of the country make it. It tasted like a cross between a cottage cheese and a store cheese. They make them in flat cakes and they are about the size of the layer in a layer cake.[4]

Gee, mother but I sure do miss those chocolate cakes you used to send me. Last Wednesday there was some mail for our outfit from the States. I did not get any. That sure was a disappointment to me. I hope that you will not disappoint me again.

I have a good place to sleep. I have all I want to eat of good, wholesome well cooked food. I have plenty of money, lots of time to myself and I am seeing the world and saving

---

4. He is describing Brie, the cheese made in the area where he was billeted.

my money. That is what the enlistment posters said. But there is one thing that I can not stand and that is being without word from home. Please write me a letter so long that it will take me an hour to read it.

We hear a lot from the front. The guns go all the time. There is no let up. The amount of money being used must be simply enormous. Aeroplanes are around and over us all the time. One gets so used to them that one does not look up to see them. You can tell by the sound whether it is a German or not so you know what you do when you hear them.

There was a place bombed about two miles from here a night or two ago. All the men who were up saw it but the rest of us just slept right on. I never heard it at all. It just goes to show how the human nature can adapt itself to any surroundings. The funny thing about it is that it is not bravery at all but simply indifference. Well, I am having a darn good time.

Letter to family, July 1, 1918

Remember I seldom see a paper anymore. We used to see them every day but we are so near the front that we do not get that kind of thing anymore. So the exciting thing of the mail airship has caused everybody to go out and look at it. I wonder if they will get tired of looking at them as we do. They have ceased to be a novelty with us. They go over us all the time. The only time we go to look at them is when there is a scrape or a bunch of about 25 or 30 go over at a time or when "Jerry" goes over. That is the American soldiers name for the Germans.

You can say there was a Pershing man there. Do you realize that this letter is from one of "Blackjack" Pershing's men? I'll tell you the boys all swear by him.

It is hard to realize that 3 days from now will be the 4th of July. It hardly seems possible that Christmas was 6 months ago and that I have been in the army almost a year.

This is about the softest thing I have struck yet. I have a good place to sleep. Plenty, yes more than I want to eat. More money than I can spend. Tobacco is issued to us. We get matches issued to us too. Nothing to worry about. Captain Fitzpatrick is a Major now. He is still commanding our outfit. Send me Simonds' articles in the Inquirer.[5]

Letter to his brother Alan, July 1, 1918

I am having a swell time. There is lots of excitement all the time but that is getting to be the ordinary thing instead of the extraordinary. I went to bed last night at about 10 o'clock and about 12 awoke and believe me, Hell sure had broke loose in France. The old building was shaking like a tree in the storm. Boy oh Boy the bombs were bursting all around us and that anti aircraft guns were popping and bursting in the air to beat the duce. The searchlights were sweeping the sky but they could not pick that Dutchman out.[6] You know there are no roads in the sky and it is a pretty big place up there and lots of clouds that an airplane can dive into and get away from us.

I had no mail from home for three or four days now. That is the only thing I can't seem to be able to get used to.

---

5. Frank H. Simonds wrote articles about World War I that were published in many newspapers. In 1919 his book *History of the World War* was published by Doubleday and Page & Co. of New York.

6. "Dutch" was a bastardization of "Deutsch" (see the glossary).

Chapter 3. France

July 4, 1918

Pierre Levee, France

Today is the anniversary of our Declaration. It is cloudy and there's no sun out at all. We are still at the Chateau. It is called the Chateau Montebise and the Villa Dauphe Oise. Americans are raising the deuce up on the line. Captured Germans are coming in all the time. Yesterday I was up to Le Ferte. Maj. Fitzpatrick is up there on official duty with the Field Hospital 23. I stopped on my way out there to see a hole by a bomb in a wheat field. It is 10 feet deep and 20 feet in diameter and the wheat is just laid flat for 50 feet around the hole like this:

Up a little further I met a batch of German prisoners who were being brought in by the French. They appeared to have enough to eat. There was one officer. He was a man about 30 years of age. Stern and sneering. The soldiers are all young none over 16. Most were young boys. Le Ferte [La Ferté] showed signs of shelling. With the exception of blowing up three or four houses nothing has been done.

Night before last we were bombed but they did not come very close to us. Lieut. Slay was at Meaux and bombs were dropped within 50 yards of the Chateau where he is quartered.

Gen. Pershing made a statement at 4th Div. Hg. that the war would

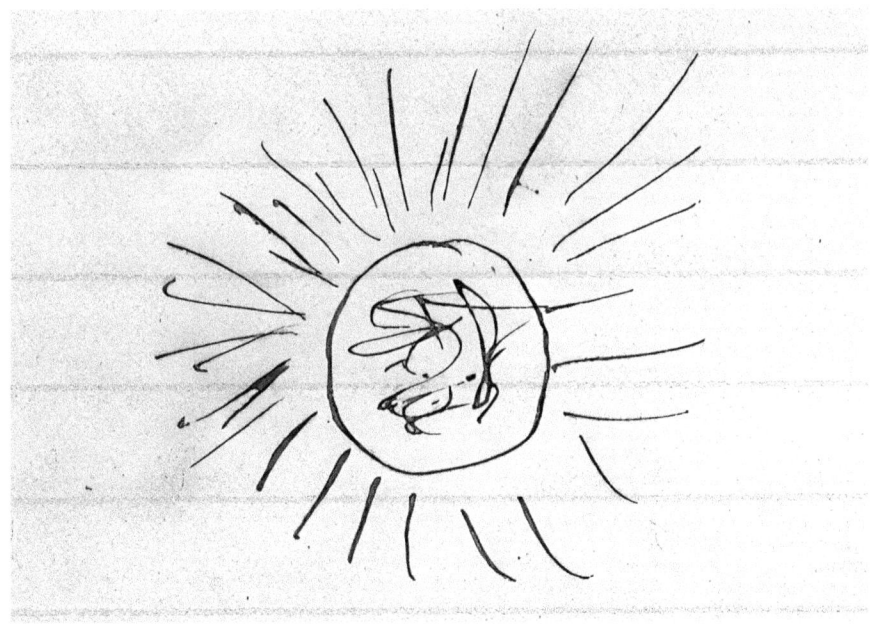

Drawing by Sergeant Brown.

be over by Christmas. That is something to look forward to. Stories are all around us about the bravery and fearlessness of the American Troops. While we were being bombed Tuesday night one of the men near me said, "Gee, I hope they don't hit the kitchen. We won't get anything to eat for a day or so."

There is a sign in the frontline trenches which says, "Soldiers are absolutely forbidden to walk on the top of this Trench." Some Sign.

There was a German officer captured the other day. He was fed. They asked him if he wanted some beef-steak. He looked at them as if he thought they were crazy. Well they gave him about a pound. It was the first he had had for months. He stated that he had been told that he would get harsh treatment if the Americans captured him. God grant that no nation ever be able to say that the United States has ever harshly treated a Prisoner of War no matter who he is or what he has done.

There was a division who took over a sector from the French just a short while ago. The Light artillery use the French 75s. When the French turned the sector over to the Americans they told us that there was enough ammunition for six months. The Americans shot it all away in 72 hours. They captured some Germans and first thing that did was to feed them. Then they asked him if there's anything else they wanted they said "yes."

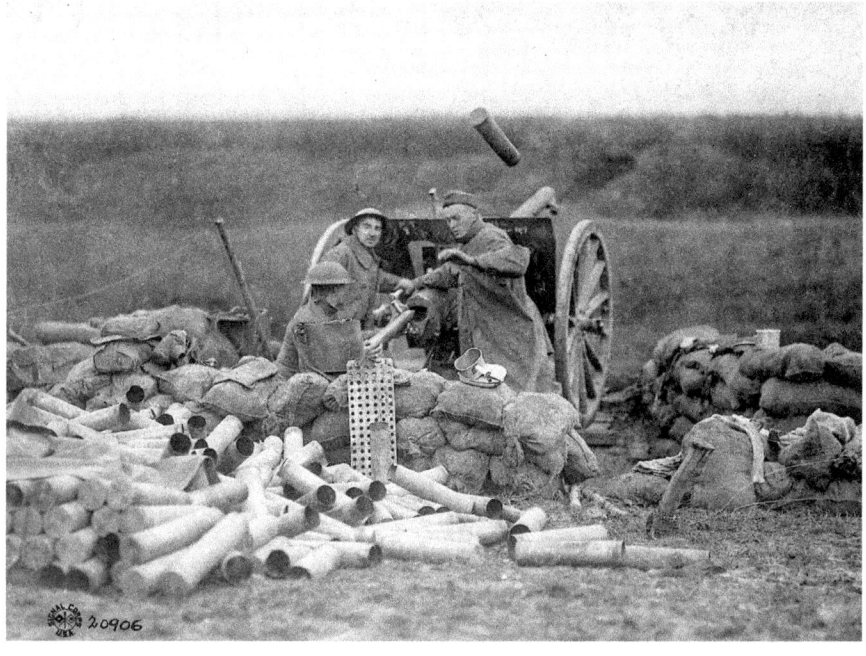

The French 75-millimeter rapid-fire cannon manned by American soldiers (Library of Congress).

Show us [the] machine gun which shoots shells. We all had a good laugh. But seriously it speaks well for our artillery.

Letter to family, July 4, 1918,

Today is the grand and glorious Fourth. We are sure hoping that it will be a day long remembered in German history as well as our own. I suppose you will read about it long before I hear anything. We have had a perfectly good night's sleep. I suppose that Jerry is going to give us a little rest but I guess the truth of the matter is that we are keeping him so busy that he doesn't have time to come over to us.

I was up a whole lot closer to the front than I have ever been. That was yesterday. I met a bunch of prisoners that had been captured. I suppose that you will read about it in yesterday's official report. Gee, but an official report is a cold, uninteresting statement. The report tells nothing at all.

I was talking to some of the men that Gen. Pershing had congratulated a day or so ago. They had the stories to tell—believe me. I will have to save them until I come back. Here is thing that I know to be true. It is all the officers can do to hold the men down to trench warfare. They want to get out and have the thing out with the Dutch. They're so anxious to fight that it is become necessary for the Commanding general to have a sign on the front line trenches: "Positively no walking on top of this trench."

The prisoners that they sent in here are sure hungry. They don't expect to get the treatment from us that they do. They said that they were told that if the Americans captured them they would be treated pretty rough. They can't understand when we give them beef steak and white bread. That is beyond all imagination for them. The first thing we do when we capture them is to feed them. Maybe they don't eat. They are not the only ones either. We do our share of that too and Uncle Sam gives us all that we want and then some. Don't worry about me.

I am alright and so far have had a peach of a time. I want to move on now and see some other part of the country. Of course I wish I could come back to the States so I could run home once in a while.

The other night when they were dropping them all around us I was with a couple of dozen men up on the roof of the building so that I could get a good view of the thing. When a bomb would explode, the remarks were funny. I don't think that anybody gave a minute of thought for his own safety. When a bomb would explode someone would say: Gee, that was a whopper, or that is closer or, it's funny they didn't get him. There was a fellow next to me and he did not say a word during the whole performance. Along about the end of it he turned and said, "Sergeant—I hope they don't hit the kitchen. We might not have any grub for a day or two." That tickled me. There he was up there in the air likely to be hit by a bomb any minute and all he could think was his grub.

We are allowed one sack of Bull Durham Tobacco every two days and now the only thing we have to buy is candy. I saw a newspaper yesterday. [I] see where you are allowed only 2 pounds of sugar a month. I feel sorry for you. I would rather be in the Army and get plenty of grub. I have had a wonderful experience and I sure do wish that Alan was old enough to be right here with me in this very same outfit. It sure would do him more good than anything else existing today.[7]

---

7. Alan is Leland's brother. He would have been 14 at this time.

July 7, 1918, Sunday

Acy-en-Multien, France

We moved by motor truck from Pierre Levee to this town last night. We evacuated our hospital patients to Field Hospital #28 at Meaux. We left Pierre Levee at 10 o'clock and got lost. There was one town that we passed through seven times. We arrived here at 5 AM. We should have been here at 2 o'clock. Hoyt went to bed and rest of the kitchen force were drunk and we were out of luck for something to eat. I lay down on the ground and slept like a log.

I have never been so tired. I had some bacon & coffee and went to the place where our office is. It is a private house and sure is [a] comfort. Germans shell this town quite often but I hope they do not take a chance at this place while we are in it.

Here's a picture of the town.

It is typical of all French towns except that this is cleaner and wider street than is generally found.

I am eating my mess at the officer's table. We had potatoes and onions out of the garden in the rear of the house.

The church shown in the picture is all shot to pieces. Repairs have been made on it but the windows have not been put in.

Here is a picture of the chap who owns the house and [it] shows our front door.

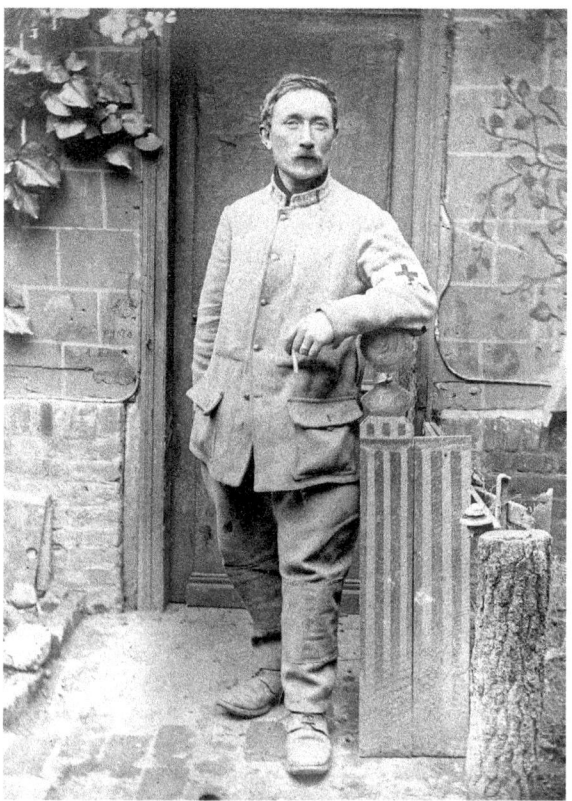

The homeowner and the house where Leland stayed in Acy-en-Multien, France. He included this photograph in his letter of July 7, 1918 (photo album).

Chapter 3. France

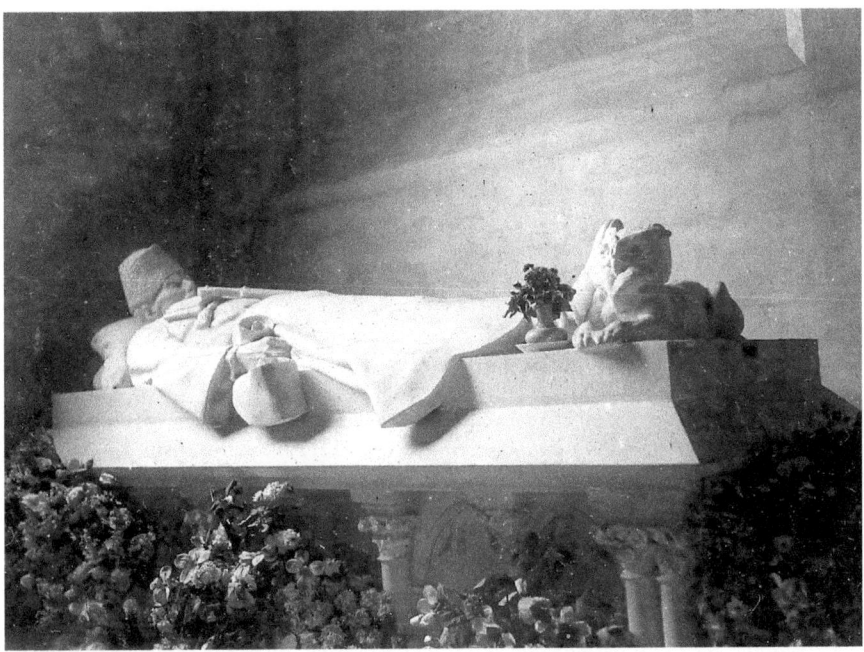

A tomb in the church across the street from the house where Sergeant Brown stayed in Acy-en-Multien, France. Leland describes the tomb in his letter of July 7, 1918, and sent this photograph along with it (photo album).

I don't know what he is leaning on. It is not here now. It must be something the Photographer carries around with him.

The picture on the other page is of a tomb in the church across the street. The supporting pillars have been partially destroyed but the main part still stands. It is a beautiful work of art. It is so lifelike that you instinctively reach out to touch the hand expecting it to move or see the chest raise and lower at each breath. The light shines down on it from the window in the roof and outlines the figure exactly as the photograph shows.

Letter to family, July 15, 1918

I am not going to say anything about the war except to say that the boys are just as anxious to put Germany out of business as they ever were.

This letter is a story of the town where we are now staying. We left our last place about a week ago and came by motor trucks here. We got lost. We left at ten and should have arrived at one but we pulled in at 5:30. We passed through our town just seven times and we never left it by the same road. It was dark and we could not make a light because the Germans see us and open fire and we could not wait until daylight because we were in a large movement of troops and we did not want the enemy to locate us.

During the night we passed the wreckage of what was once an ammunition train.[8] *It was right at the crossroads and it was supposed that they stopped and used a flashlight to read the signboard. Every man was wiped out and all the ammunition destroyed. The trucks were battered and blown all over the place and a hole was dug in the road deep enough to bury four, two-story houses.*

We traveled over one of the finest pieces of road that I have ever had the pleasure of riding over. The Romans taught the French the art of building roads and the French have learned their lesson well. The particular piece of road in front of the house [where] I am now living was built by Napoleon Bonaparte and four years of war and travel and heavy guns and trucks and tanks traveling over it have failed to put it out of commission. I think that some of our road builders should come over and learn a lesson or two. The roads are lined with poplars. Those tall lean trees [are] always in pairs. The tops touch and the trees from each side of the road lean in and at night remind me of two whispering people.

Now the town [is] typical of all French towns you will ever see or read about. The streets are sometimes narrow and sometimes wide. Dirty and never clean. Sometimes the houses are built out over the sidewalk and often the corner sticks out into the street. Other times, and as [in] the case of the place where I am living, a wall runs all around the house and grounds. It is built right where the sidewalk would be and is about 6 feet high. It is an ugly wall-white and tumbled down. [You enter] through a little tiny gate and then you walk into sort of [a] courtyard. On the right is the stable and a cow shed and on the left is a woodpile and the manure dump. The rest of the yard is or was a dirty dump. The house-well to look at it from the outside you would think it was a part of the stable, but step in. First comes two little rooms all apart by themselves. These were a chemist laboratory.[9] *In the living room (our office) [is] also my bedroom. I have a mattress which I sleep on. During the day I roll it up and put it in a closet. The room itself-an open fireplace, an ordinary window and a door which is a window leading out into the garden in the back of the house; a sideboard, made of dark oak and covered with hand carved figures. Soft easy chairs which are too modern to describe. The floor is made of blocks of stone. Next-the dining room-a small narrow room built to eat meals and for no other purpose. The dishes and chinaware are still here. I can't write well enough to describe them. Then the kitchen—a fairly large room, an open fireplace for cooking and also a modern range for cooking. The second floor contains beds, but to get from one room to another it is necessary to walk through the rest of the rooms. I don't see how the French have any privacy at all.*

The bedrooms are occupied by officers. In back of the house is the garden. Potatoes, peas, string beans, rhubarb, lettuce, turnips. We sure do feed. We get meals and coffee and best of all real, American whole wheat bread. We used to get French shoe leather but now we get real bread.

Tuesday 2 PM p.m. July 16, 1918

Acy-en-Multien

Last night will live in my memory as long as I live. I had the pleasure

---

8. An ammunition train is a convoy of trucks and/or wagons carrying ammunition.
9. "Chemist" is another word for "pharmacist."

Chapter 3. France 59

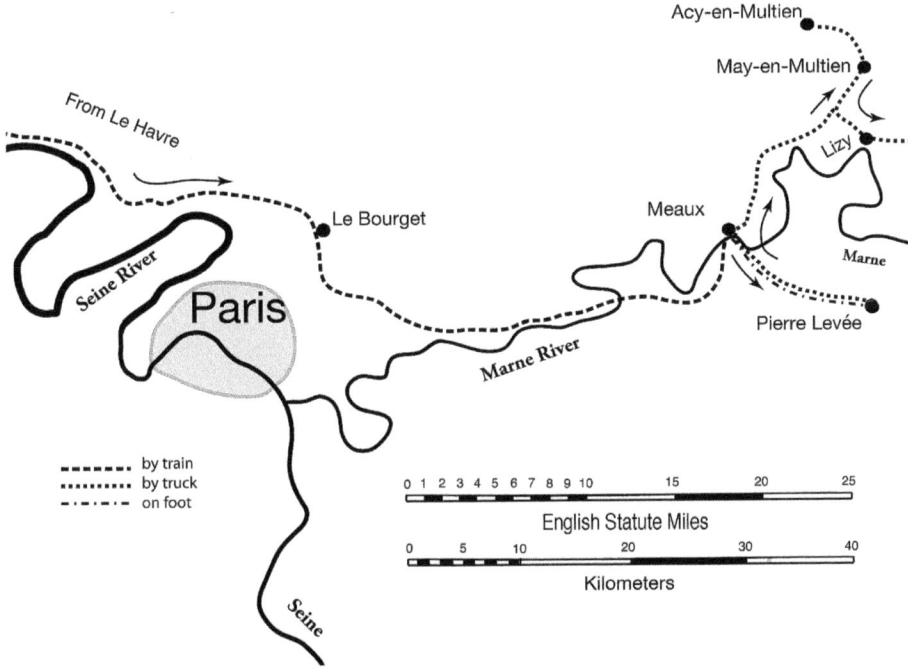

Le Bourget is where Sergeant Brown met the young French soldier Jean Cherfils. See the appendix for additional information about Cherfils.

After landing at Le Havre on June 12, 1918, Sergeant Brown traveled on June 14 by train to Meaux and arrived there the next day. On the way to Meaux, their train stopped at Le Bourget, where he met the French soldier Jean Cherfils. From Meaux on that same day he and his company marched to Pierre-Levée, a distance of about nine miles.

On July 6, Sergeant Brown and his outfit, Field Hospital No. 33, motored by truck to Acy-en-Multien.

Then, on July 16, Sergeant Brown drove with a friend in a Model T ambulance to Coupru (their route is denoted on this map by a dotted line). At Coupru he vividly described the beginning of the Aisne-Marne Offensive by the AEF and its allies (map by author).

of witnessing one of the famous German drives. Let me say that there is always the expectation of the big attack. Sometimes it comes and sometimes not. We are located about 10 km from a direct line from Chateau Thierry to Paris.[10] There has been signs of a drive on this front for the last two weeks. Yesterday morning the Germans began shelling Meaux with

---

10. When he says, "We are located about 10 km. from a direct line from Paris to Château Thierry," he means that Acy-en-Multien is 10 kilometers from the road that runs from Paris to Château-Thierry.

their long range gun. A shell was just put in the town every 10 minutes from 6 AM to 11 AM. All day there was an intense artillery preparation from Chateau Thierry to Reims so last night I decided to go over to have a look at the battle. I am going to write the official report and then try to tell what I saw.

Official:—

After a violent preparation with artillery, the Germans, attacked from Chateau Thierry to Reims. Our troops are energetically withstanding the enemy's shock. East of Chateau Thierry a vigorous counter-attack by our troops drove the enemy out of their positions.

The battle is still continuing.

Unofficial:—

I jumped into one of Henry Ford's ambulances and took the road from Acy [Acy-en-Multien] to Rosoy [Rosoy-en-Multien] to May [May-en-Multien]. Then the main Paris Road to Lizy. Then from Lizy to Cocherel to La Ferto [La Ferté] Road which runs direct to the Chateau [Château-Thierry]. Straight to a little crossroads to Coupru. There we left

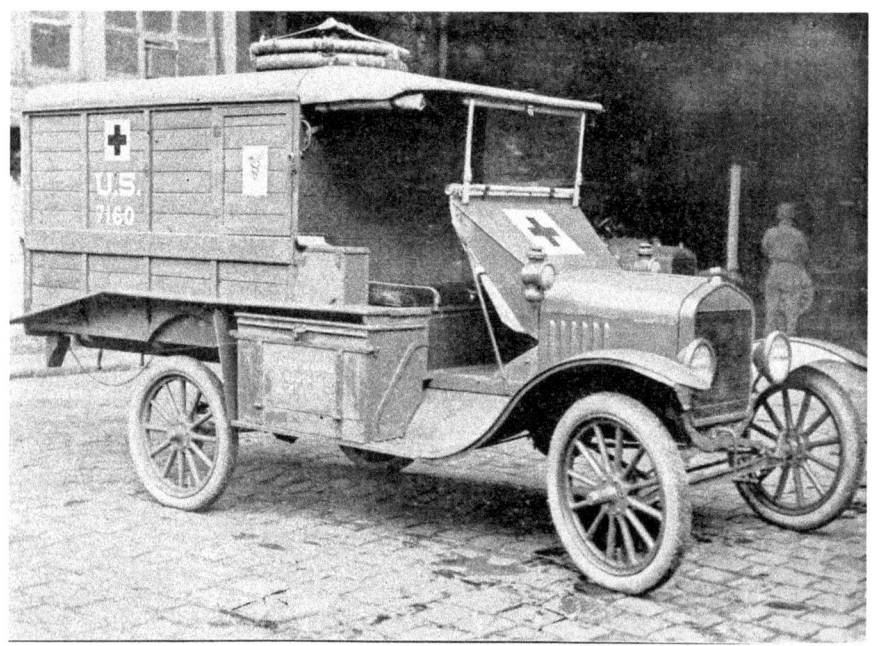

World War I Model T Ford ambulance. Sergeant Brown's route on a Model T ambulance is shown on the map before his 2 p.m. diary entry of July 16, 1918 (*The Medical Department of the United States Army in the World War*, Vol. VIII, fig. 44).

Chapter 3. France

the machine and proceeded to an artillery emplacement near hill 208. We were then on high ground 3 miles from Vaux and 4 miles from the from the town of Chateau Thierry. We were high in the air and the battle line was laid out in front of us like [a] map.[11]

Shell[s] were bursting around the hill all the time. We soon were able to tell when a shell passed over whether it was one of our own or a German. The infantry could be seen by the fire of the rifles. When we arrived at the hill it was about 12:30 [a.m.]. The Germans had just finished an artillery preparation on the American lines held by the 26th Division and they were just going over the top. No man's land was as light as day because of the Very lights and Star Shells.[12]

The Germans could be seen advancing. They came first in extended order. These would be wiped out by our machine guns. Then more extended order. Then more. Very few lived to even get near our barbed wire. Then came the real infantry advance. They came over the top in that massed formation. Oh Hell sure broke loose then. Machine guns. Infantry fire and artillery. How any man could ever live through that rain of steel and iron I don't know but they did manage to reach our trenches. They poured in and poured in like water from a pump to a pitcher and all the time machine guns and artillery kept up. Down there those men were fighting hand to hand. No bullets, just cold steel. The Germans sure hate that. Then our artillery and machine guns quit. No heavy firing except on the German side and then our guns broke out again and out of the American trenches went the Dutch with the Americans after them.

Just at this time we heard a terrific explosion on the other side of the hill. Went over and found the gun had been blown up. A direct hit for the Germans. We found only two men. One was dead. The other had his leg blown of[f] above the knee and his body was just peppered with little wounds. We put a tourniquet on him and rubbed him up with iodine and put on some bandages and beat it to the Field Hospital at Coupru with him. We had no litter but we made one out of two poles and an overcoat.

That finished that night for us. We got back to my quarters at 5 o'clock. I have only told a small fraction of the things I saw. I can't remember it all. We wore our gas masks all the time we were up there. While we were walking from Coupru we had a peculiar experience of going down

---

11. This was the beginning of the Aisne-Marne offensive, which was also known as the Second Battle of the Marne, in which the Germans believed that an attack through Flanders would give them a decisive victory, but that attack was repelled by the British and the Americans.

12. Very (or Verey) lights are flares. Star shells are incendiary shells that are used for lighting and not for arson purposes. The star shell is shot up and descends slowly by a parachute. The image (I believe) shows star shells.

a road under shell fire. That gives you the funniest feeling. To be walking down the road and have a shell burst about ½ mile away. Then one a little closer-than close. Boy, oh boy your hair stands on end then if it ever did before and you think of all your sins and you can't remember a nice thing you ever did in your life and all the mean things you have done come up in a lump and you can't forget them.

Man dear, but you think of the loved ones [at] home too.[13]

We have our hospital running and receiving American Wounded from the 4th Division—The 39th Infantry seems to be having the most casualties.

Letter to family, July 18, 1918

The war is coming along fine. We are going to lick the Dutch and they know it. This new offensive is showing them that Uncle Sammy's boys are the real thing. This offensive is only three days old now. Last night they came over in aeroplanes and bombed this town. One of the shells broke in our back yard but the only military damage it did was to blow up some of the potato patch. So we did not have any potatoes for supper. It is now 10 o'clock and I am going to sit up for a couple of hours to see the fun. Germany is going to yell for peace pretty soon.

There is not much happening around here just now except a battle and I can't tell you about that. Wait until I get back home I'll tell you the tales. It has been almost 2 months since I sailed. I never knew time to pass so quickly. Thanks for the papers. A good American paper is a rare article here. Be sure and have the number of the post office on my mail in the future. A.P.O. means American post office. That is all the news I can find in this letter so I'll quit now and go out and watch the battle.

Editor's Note: The Aisne-Marne Offensive, July 28–August 6, 1918

In late July of 1918, the 4th Division was withdrawn from the French Sixth Army (with whom they had been fighting) and became solely part of the AEF. They then became part of the Army's First Corps.

The Germans had begun attacks east and west of the city of Reims. On the east they had little success, but on the west the Germans advanced about four miles across the Marne river.

The German salient (bulge) at one point had reached from the southern side of the Marne to Soissons in the north and to Château-Thierry in the south.

---

13. Supposedly there was a deception planted by the Allies. A briefcase with false plans for an American counterattack was handcuffed to a man who had died of pneumonia and placed in a vehicle that appeared to have run off the road at a German-controlled bridge. The Germans, on finding him and being taken in by these plans, adjusted their attack to thwart the false Allied plan. Consequently, the French and American forces were able to unleash a different attack on the exposed parts of the enemy lines, leaving the Germans with no choice but to retreat.

Chapter 3. France

On the night of August 1–2, the 4th Division, to which Sergeant Brown and Field Hospital No. 33 belonged, moved into Fôret de Fere and attempted to take over the ground that was held by the 42nd Division of the AEF. On August 3 they held a line running east to west though the middle of the Fôret de Nesles. During that night and the next day, the division advanced to the southern bank of the Vesle river, where they met with heavy German resistance. During their retreat, the Germans left well-concealed and strategically placed machine gun nests to slow the advancing of American troops.

On the night of August 4–5 a small number of the 4th Division soldiers crossed the Vesle, but their progress was arduous and slow. Without proper artillery support, those who did cross had to retreat.

The rapid advancement of the 4th Division made it difficult to provide proper care to the sick and wounded. On August 3, Field Hospital No. 33—along with two other field hospitals, No. 19 and No. 21—were ordered to Épaux-Bézu. Field Hospitals No. 33 and No. 19 opened for the sick and the seriously wounded, while Field Hospital No. 21 was held in reserve. Field Hospital No. 28 was moved six kilometers closer to the front at Bezu–Saint-Germain to specifically treat gas patients. These four field hospitals were all part of the 4th Division's Sanitary Train.

Because of poor weather, deplorable road conditions, and lack of enough transport, dressing stations were expanded into a triage.

As the advance became stalled and the casualties became more numerous, specially constructed shock rooms and a station for the slightly wounded were established. War neuroses were attended to by the division psychiatrist in a separate ward. At this station the wounded were moved to the proper field hospital.

Due to the hilly terrain of the area of battle, removal of the wounded was difficult. This was delayed until nightfall, so as to avoid exposure to the enemy.

On August 6, the field hospitals were relocated to Château de la Fôret, where they were well concealed by the surrounding forest. In addition to the experienced personnel who were part of the four field hospitals at Château de la Fôret, three additional surgical teams, two shock teams, and seven additional nurses were also on-site. A portable X-ray machine was brought to the château. Field Hospital No. 19 used the château for those wounded who could not be moved. On the château grounds, ward tents were erected for the other field hospitals: Field Hospital No. 33 treated sick patients, No. 21 was for neurological patients, and No. 28 was for those who had been gassed. Triage was established there as well. The result was that a complete center was established for the treatment of the sick and wounded.

At Château de la Fôret, the 4th Division's field hospitals were in a reasonably secure location. Because of this, the personnel were able to work unhindered from the nervous strain and fear of being shelled or gassed. They were located on a good road with decent access to the front.

The advantages of reducing the number of care-giving personnel and the efficiency of treating the wounded by the grouping of field hospitals became apparent. Certain parameters were recommended for battlefield treatment of the wounded: ensure no fewer than 100 trained medical personnel for each regiment of 6,500 men; replace the aid stations at the front with dressing stations provided by an ambulance company; increase the number and quality of the motor transports of the wounded; treat shock patients with properly trained personnel before evacuation by keeping them warm, resting them, and providing morphine as required; provide proper treatment of the gassed by bathing them at the battalion aid station or the dressing station; and place the field hospitals as far forward as possible despite the potential of greater danger.

Due to the poor sanitary facilities that the 4th Division experienced from August 1 to August 12, nearly 80 percent of the personnel contracted gastroenteritis.

On August 11–12, the 4th Division was relieved by the 77th Division, and on August 14 it moved to training stations near Montmirail and then to the area of Rimaucourt for rest, relaxation, and training.[14]

July 20, 1918, Saturday

Acy-en-Multien

We are very busy handling American wounded. I suppose this battle will be known as the battle of Soissons Heights. For the past week orders have been sent out to us and all preparations were made for the troops on this part of the line to retreat. In fact orders were sent to this effect. This was done purposefully so that the German[s] would think we were prepared to get out and that we were expecting an attack.

The Germans did exactly what was wanted of them. They did not attack on this sector but did attack at Chateau Thierry. The result was that this part of the line was weak and in as much as the Germans thought we were about to retreat, he was not expecting us and when we did attack it sure was a surprise.

---

14. Charles Lynch, Frank W. Weed, and Loy McAfee, eds., *The Medical Department of the United States Army in the World War*, Vol. VIII (Washington, D.C.: U.S. Army Surgeon General's Office, 1923–29) 400–403.

I have talked to some captured Germans; one fellow said, "Thank God it is all over for him because there is nothing for them to eat in Germany."

Others remain haughty and refused to talk.

Some are afraid we are going to kill them, one fellow said, "At last I believe the Americans are here."

Another one asked if we were English or French. He does not believe that we are Americans. [He] thinks we are just dressed in American uniforms.

The battle was in the open yesterday. The 39th advanced over the old German territory. The advance was during a gas attack. While they were in it they met the German infantry. A Sergeant told me that he could not see well through his mask. He could not tell whether he was fighting American, French or German. He saw a fellow trying to bayonet an American. He went for him but the American did not have his bayonet fixed and did not realize it until he tried to use it. The result was he was up against it. He struck the German by throwing his gun at him. This gave him a chance to get his revolver [out] and one shot was enough to finish the German.

Shell shock is a funny thing. A Captain was brought into us suffering with it. He had fought and captured 11 Germans. He was bringing them back when a high explosive shell went off about 20 feet away. He was picked up and brought to us. There was not a mark on the body. He came around but he is nutty as a loon. Yesterday his nurse found him creeping out of the tent. He wore his helmet, his gas mask in the alert position and he was carrying his shoes in his hand.

We have two American Red Cross women assigned to us. They are two freaks of nature. Maj. Fitzpatrick calls them "American Nuts." He refuses to have anything to do with them. He will not even eat his meal if they are at the table.[15]

Letter to family, July 23, 1918

I received two copies of the Sunday Inquirer. The boys read everything in those papers—even the women's section. There is a special mess for the noncoms and that is where it costs me money. Not much and yet I can soon spend a lot there if I wish. With the grub the government furnishes plus what we buy, a fellow can live like a king. I have quite a few remembrances of France. I hope I can get to some large city in the south of France so I can send you a few little trinkets. As for going to Paris, it is a forbidden city to all soldiers unless on official business.

---

15. The Second Battle of the Marne was an important victory. The Allies had taken 29,367 prisoners, 793 guns, and 3,000 machine guns and inflicted 168,000 casualties on the Germans. The primary importance of the battle was its morale aspect: the strategic gains on the Marne marked the end of a string of German victories and the beginning of a series of Allied ones that would in three months cause the German army to surrender (source: *Wikipedia*).

Letter to family, July 24, 1918

Received your letter of July 2. The map was in there and I have been wanting a map of France ever since I came here. Tell anyone that leaves for France to be sure bring a map with them. It does not do them any good except that when they hear that the Allies have taken a town they can tell where it is. Is also gives you a good idea all the places you have been. You are allowed to tell where you are or where you have been provided you are not in the front line. But that is where I have been almost all the time since I have been in France. The regulation was made so that men going on a furlough could tell the folks at home that they have visited a certain town.

Yesterday Major Fitzpatrick was up on the line. He was about a half kilometer from where the fighting was going on. The closest that any of our men have been as yet. The fighting is all out in the open and it is every man for himself. He said that the German dead were scattered all over the place. Those that have been captured and who have passed through our hands all seemed glad that they are out of it. They all tell the same story that there is nothing for them to eat. I wish you could see them go for the white bread that was handed them at the first aid station. When I was in the States I could look forward to a pass once in a while but now I can only see 3 more years over here. We may, and no doubt will be kept over here for a year or more after the war is over to look after the sick and the wounded that are left. The returning prisoners will be some job if all the reports that are circulated are true. I don't think that the Germans worry much about their prisoners. I have talked to several men who have been prisoners in Germany and they do not want to repeat the experience.

Letter to family, July 30, 1918

We have moved again. It suits me to a T. It would suit me if we kept right on going to Berlin. I am quartered in a little town right behind the lines. It was captured from the Germans in this last drive. Last night I went out on the battlefield to see the old trenches. The dead are still lying out there unburied. Our men are over [there] digging graves for the Americans and when that is done they will bury the Dutch. German equipment is scattered all over the place. We are near one of the roads and prisoners are passing thru all the time.

I get a daily paper (New York Herald) every day. It is published in Paris and we get it about 10 o'clock in the morning. It contains all the official dope about the war but none of the home news. That is what I want. I have not read all the Record yet but as soon as I get through with one I pass it along to Lt. Dick or some of the other Phila. boys.[16]

I read in one of the papers of one Yankee Soldier who went into the German [lines] and got lost and was captured by some Germans. He told them they were surrounded and they surrendered to him and led them to his own lines. Genl. Pershing gave him the D.S.M. for it. I was talking to this man's commanding officer on Sunday. He told me the story like this.

The soldier was a cook. Cooks have every other day off. So this cook took his day off and proceeded to celebrate by getting drunk. On this way back to camp he got lost and wandered over to the German lines where he was promptly captured. He had two bottles of wine with him and these he shared with the Germans. He could speak a little Spanish and German and they could speak a little Spanish and English. Soon the Germans and the American began to get pretty drunk and both ended up by boasting of how much better their army was than the other fellow's. The German told how good his

---

16. *The Philadelphia Record* was a newspaper.

army was. The American said, "Why you fellow[s] are you so d____ dumb you don't know you are alive. Why you are surrounded now and in a half an hour you all will be dead men." The German carried this news to his officer. They talked it over and decided to give themselves up and told the American to take them back. He told them he did not know the way and they said they would show him. Well they did. Our sentries halted him and asked him who went there. He said one American and the whole German Army. When he came in sight he was walking in the lead. He had a sword in one hand and a wine bottle in the other. He gravely saluted this sentry with the sword and marched them to the Battalion Headquarters. That is how he won his D.S.M.[17]

July 31, 1918

Wednesday
Bouresches, France
We moved here on the 29th. This town was held by the Germans on 14th of July. Their trenches were just beyond here and are not the deep type but narrow shallow ditches.

Letter to family, August 3, 1918

I moved quite often in the past week. The Germans are going back so fast that it keeps us busy pulling up stakes and following them. What men who are not busy in the hospital are digging graves for the German dead. It is a job and a problem to get rid of the bodies. I went out for a walk the other night and saw hundreds of unburied Germans. I saw one fellow still sitting behind a machine gun.

Day before yesterday I passed through one of the large French towns which was the closest point the Germans were to Paris in their drive of June 6th.[18] Things are pretty well shot up but not so bad as the towns which are nearer the line. These are completely destroyed. I saw a shell hole which was 30 feet in diameter and 20 feet deep. It was right alongside an important road but it missed the mark and was wasted.

August 5.
Had to move my office again and could not finish my letter to you. I think one letter a week is a bum idea. Please try to make it 3 or 4. We move almost every day.

---

17. As reported in the American papers, Frank P. Lennart described how, on July 2, he was forced to capture 83 Germans near Belleau Woods: "You see, I got caught between lines and discovered a machine gun staring straight at me, and dived into a shell hole."
Lennart slowly raised his head and saw that the German didn't shoot. After Lennart assured him that they were surrounded, the gunner conveyed that he and others wanted to surrender. Lennart told him that they should before they were killed. The German agreed and requested that he take them to the Americans.
They all walked with their hands raised but got lost. Finally they found an American sentry who was surprised to see them. Other American soldiers came up to help him, but Lennart insisted that he take them to headquarters as it was "...his party."
(Source: *The Cherokee Harmonizer* (Center, Alabama), July 4, 1918)
In the records of the soldiers who were awarded the Distinguished Service Medal, Lennart's name was not found.
18. Probably Château-Thierry

The line going forward so fast that it keeps us on the jump all the time. We have had lots of rain in the past six or seven days. It can rain all it wants for then the aeroplanes can not come out and bomb us.

Maj. Fitzpatrick is going to Paris in a few days to open a bank account. He has promised to take me. We can run down there in a few hours in the machine. The roads are good all the way.

Letter to family, August 9, 1918

I received Dad's letter dated July 21. When I first received it I could not understand what the funny stamp was. First I thought that the postal rates have been raised and then after I looked at it a while I saw that it had been sent to New York by the Air Mail service.[19] That letter sure was quick in getting here. I was quite surprised that you knew we were in the big drive. I have written and told you some about it but of course only a small bit. Our boys are simply great. Everybody over here hands it to them. I was talking to a German last night. He had just been captured, was wounded and in our hospital. I felt sorry for the poor devil. He was scared stiff. He said that at first they were told that the Americans did not amount to much but now they were told to be very careful of the Americans, that they were more treacherous than the English. This particular German was afraid that the Americans would not treat him right in the hospital and was going to have some devilish way of killing him.

The French too give the Americans a lot of credit for the victory. I have a souvenir of the battle. I am going to send home a German helmet. I will do it as soon as I can go to a post office. It is about 25 miles from where I am now but one of these days I am going to get there and I will send it.

I have been over most of the territory that has been recaptured from the Germans. One thing that surprised me most is how quickly roads and railroads are repaired. How quickly bridges are made or repaired. This is surely an efficient army.

Now about the terrible destruction you see on the battlefield. Big cannon and little cannon and quantities of ammunition are abandoned by the retreating armies just as you read in the papers. Personal equipment is scattered all over the fields. That shows that the Germans left in a hurry. The trenches that you find around here are little narrow ditches just big enough to shelter one man. The artillery too was out in the open. The fields are potted with shell holes.

(I just stopped my letter to go out and look at a German plane which was trying to pass the lines. He passed them and I can hear him now. He is in a big cloud which is over us. He is flying around up there but we can't see him. I hear an Allied plane up there but I can't see them. There goes the anti-aircraft guns again. I can't hear the planes now. It doesn't take them that long to get away. He must have been after some of the observation balloons. It is just an incident in the days work.)

Now to go back to my letter. The woods are not as much shot up as you would think. All branches are shot off up to the height of the man's head. There are quite a number of trees shot down but the damage is not as great as you would think it would be.

---

19. Regularly scheduled airmail service by the U.S. Postal Service was instituted on May 15, 1918, between Washington and New York, stopping in Philadelphia. The original postage was 24 cents per ounce but was lowered to 16 cents on July 15, 1918. The lower rate was perhaps an incentive for Leland's father to send him an airmail letter. (Source: "Airmail: A Brief History," https://about.usps.com/who-we-are/postal-history/airmail.pdf)

Chapter 3. France

The woods are filled with dead horses. It doesn't smell very nice. Can you imagine an immense boneyard? Well that is what the new battlefield smells like. The part of the country which is hardest hit is [are] the towns. All that is left is a few brick walls. Beautiful houses and churches shot up like a pile of bricks. These are the places that remind you that a war is really is going on.

The German aeroplane came back. Three American planes are coming. They are going over my head now. There will be one less Fritz aviator in a minute or two. There go their machine guns. They're climbing up now. I'll go on with my letter.

The wounded who come here have lots of tales to tell but there is a wonderful thing about them. You never hear them groan or say a word about their troubles.

Last night I was in an ambulance. We had to pass a place in the road that was under shell fire. A shell would come over and burst and then we would scoot for the other end of the road. It certainly was an exciting minute. If you don't believe me come over here and do it and you will find out.

There was a regiment camped near here last night. I took a walk and who should meet but Forbes. He talked for quite a while and today at noon he came over to the hospital and had dinner with me. His outfit is going to Paris for a 6 weeks rest. I bet they don't do much resting. I know I would not if I was given permission to go see that city. Did I tell you that I saw the Eiffel tower and the spires of that famous church in Paris? I saw them from the railroad while we were passing.

I have read the Record all right. It sure is great to pick up a newspaper and read a couple of columns about something you have been in. You can bet that I am anxious to see what the papers in the States are saying about the big drive we are in.

I have seen some of the famous German concrete pill boxes. Some are small things only big enough for one man and a machine gun. And some are big enough for dozens. It looks exactly like the pictures you see of them in the papers.

August 10 Saturday

We are at a place near Fere-en Tardenois. Quite a lot is happening since I wrote last. Just as I started to write in the diary at Boureches we received orders to move to Epaux. We packed and went and arrived about 10 AM, August 1. While we were at Bouresches I walked out over the wheat fields and thru Belleau Woods. They're certainly shot up. There is a railroad which has been blown up about every 10 feet.

The woods are full of graves. American Marines, French and Germans. Lots of Germans, American Marines and French were still unburied. We buried a lot of the Americans. We did not have time to bury the Germans or the French. The place sure did stink. There was one place where we buried five Marines. The bodies were very much decomposed. The only way to get the bodies in the graves was to take three shovels. Put one under the head, one under the body and one under the legs and have the three men lift together. We were not wise to how to get the bodies into the graves and two of the boys picked up a fellow up, one on the shoulders and one on the feet. The dead man fell apart in the middle.

I saw a dead German here too. He was killed by a high explosive shell. His feet, or rather his toes, were sticking up in the air. His body was laying with the stomach on the ground. His face was turned toward the sky. He still had his helmet on but his head was smashed to a pulp. One arm was shot off and he stunk like a very, very dead horse. He was buried by simply piling dirt over him.

The trenches here are like the big ones only in the fact that they connect with each other. They are very narrow and not very deep. When I saw them on 31st of July they still had abandoned equipment in them. Overcoats, Dead, Hand grenades and machine gun belts and bullets and cartridges.[20]

The place at Epaux was pretty nice. When we got there the Germans were still at Fere-en Tardenois. The evening of August 1 was clear. A fine night for an air raid. Raid they did—I slept on the second floor. I just got laid down when there was some explosion in the front yard. Before I could get out of bed there were two more explosions. All night long this kept up but I managed to get a good night's sleep. We are in a place where the road [is] an important point in our communications. It ran around the chateau like this:

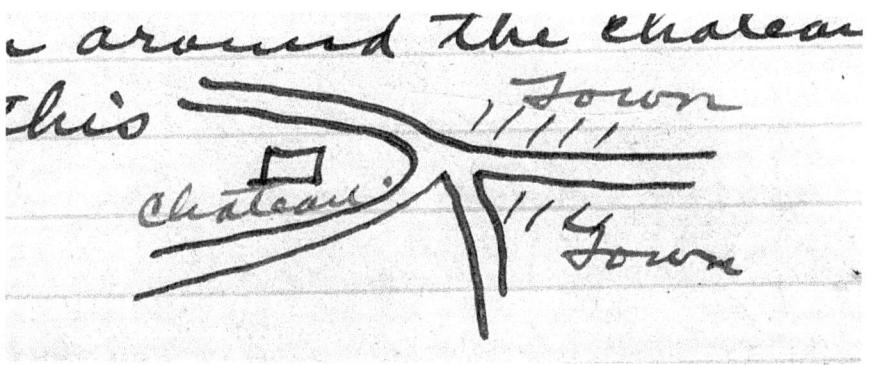

A sketch that Sergeant Brown made in his diary of the Château de la Forêt. This château was used by Field Hospital No. 33 for the seriously wounded (photo album).

---

20. The Battle of Belleau Wood was a series of battles that took place from June 6 through June 26 of 1918 with heavy casualties on both sides. At one point the battle consisted of a treacherous advance by the American Marine Corps across an open wheat field defended by machine guns on both sides. Consequently, the casualties suffered on June 6 were the highest in Marine Corps history. The woods were retaken by the Germans and then captured by the A.E.F. a total of six times before the Allies finally succeeded in driving out the Germans.

U.S. forces suffered 9,777 casualties, of which 1,811 were fatal. An unknown number of Germans were killed, but 1,600 were taken prisoner. The Battle at Belleau Wood ended on June 26, and Sergeant Brown and his detail were just burying the dead on August 1. The bodies must have been there for 35 days or longer.

The Germans were trying to block up that road but they did not hit the road, but they almost put an end to the chateau. Every day after that until we left it rained but this did not worry the Germans. They kept bombarding us with high explosives.

We found an unexploded aireal [sic] torpedo on the front lawn about 25 feet from one of our ward tents.

We left Epaux on the 6th and arrived at this place on the same day. I forgot to say that while I was at Epaux I went to one of the Q.M.C. Depots for some tents. We passed through Chateau Thierry. It is certainly a wrecked place. The houses are still standing. They have their roofs on and that is all you can say for them. I passed through Vaux too. It is some shot up place too. The streets are clean and all the debris has been removed from the side walks.

Well I saw the German pillboxes. They look exactly like the pictures you see of them.

Chateau Thierry is in a valley and the hills around it are covered with these pill boxes.

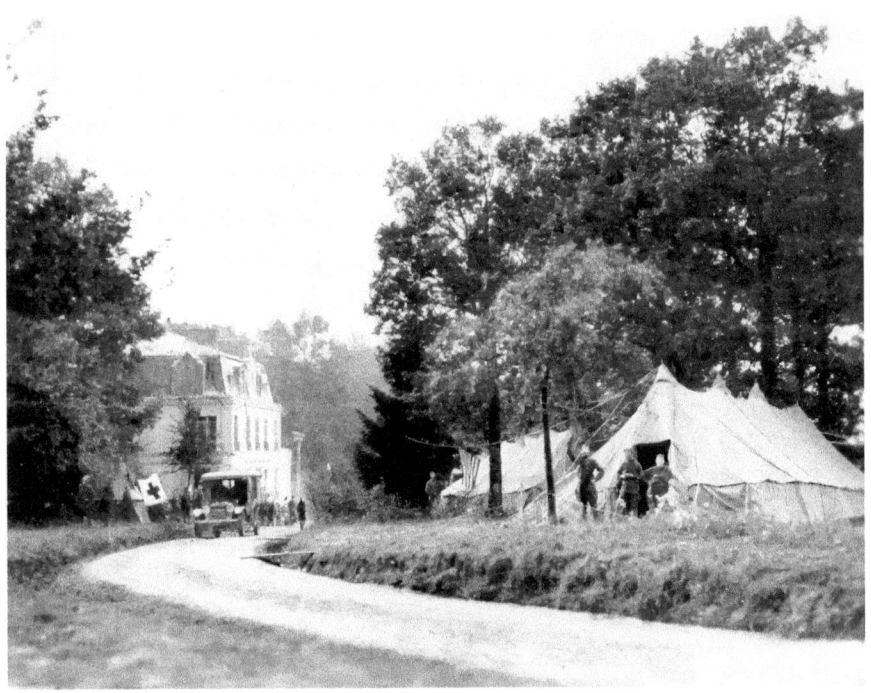

Field hospitals of the 4th Division (Sergeant Brown's division) at Château de la Forêt, August 10, 1918 (*The Medical Department of the U.S. Army in the World War*, Vol. XIII, fig. 60).

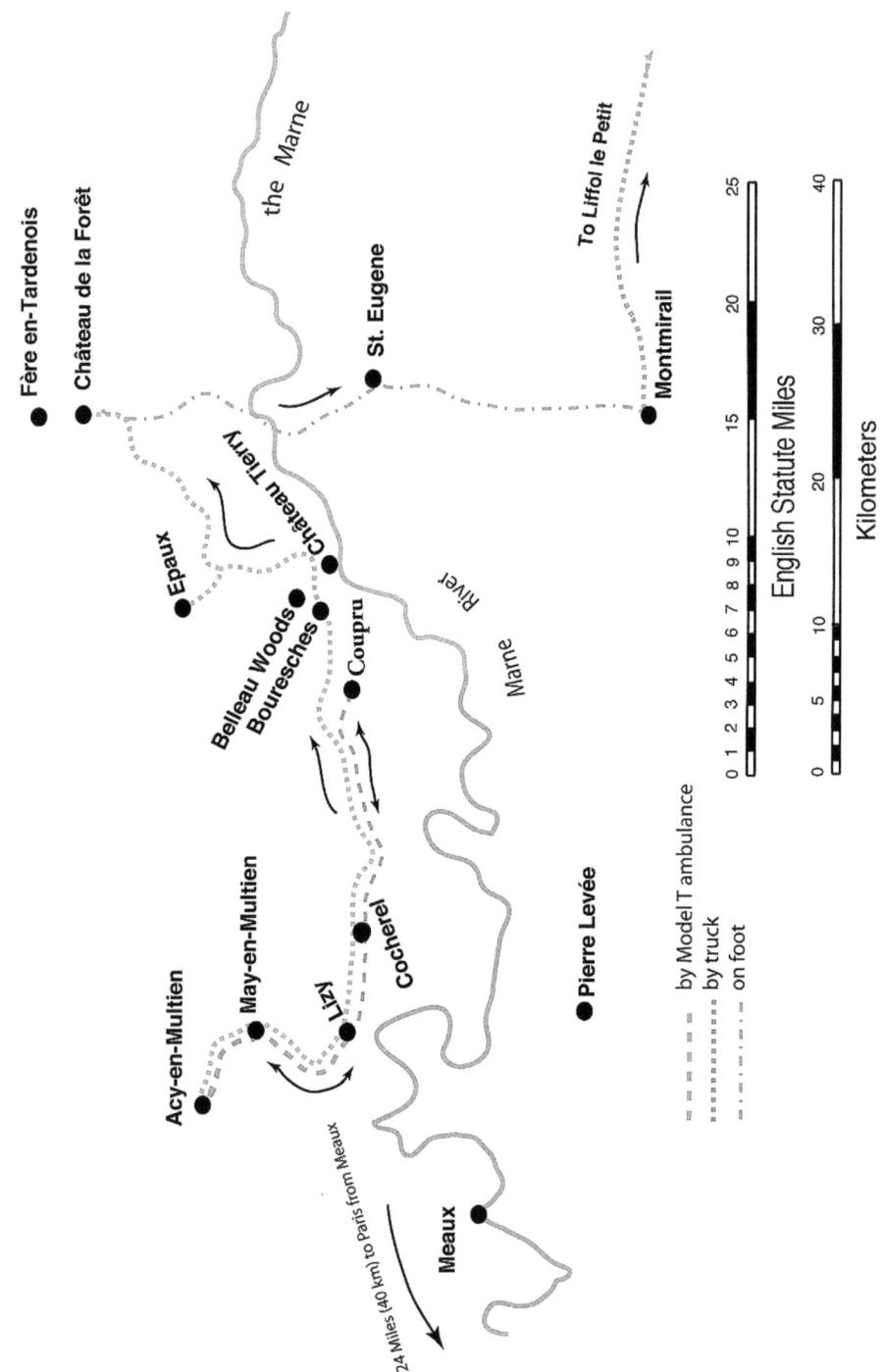

Chapter 3. France

Now about our new place. It is, or was, the dirtiest place I have ever struck yet. Dead men and horses laid all of the place. We buried them all and the place smells better now. Every night the Germans shell us and the town of Fere-en Tardenois with high explosives. We had to pass a place which was under continuous fire, a shell would strike and then we would make a run for the other end of the road before the next shell would strike. It certainly was an exciting half minute. I don't recommend it for anyone with a weak heart.

Night before last I took a little walk and ran into Forbes. Gee but Cliff was glad to see me. We talked for a couple of hours and swapped tales. He is with the 169th Infantry Rainbow Division. They are the men who stopped the Prussian guards. Yesterday he came over and ate dinner with me.

Today we burned a lot of rubbish. There was a lot of live ammunition and the bullets kept us busy all the time. There was an inspection—Colonel Carswell, Major Wilmerding & Major Bethea. There was a British Colonel with them.

Had a letter from Dad yesterday. Sent by the Air Mail service. He said that he knew our division was in the drive.

Monday 12 August 1918

We are still at Chateau De La Foret. Two months ago I landed in France and altho I have written Marian about two letters a week since I arrived, I have not heard from her. Perhaps the following clipping explains it. You never can tell[21]:

Letter to family, August 13, 1918

I read the Sunday Inquirer[s] for July 14–21 [faint]. We are going away from the line for rest somewhere and now I will have something to read for a day or two. I noticed an

---

21. A clipping in the diary tells of many girls back home who'd found other men. It was a hard time for Sergeant Brown. He had left for overseas on May 26 and hadn't heard from his girlfriend, Marian, for over 78 days. He didn't get a letter from her until September 11—108 days after he sailed from New York.

Opposite: On August 1, Sergeant Brown, along with Field Hospital No. 33, moved from Bouresches to Épaux. Three days later they relocated to Marœuil. On August 6 the company moved to Château de la Forêt. They remained there until August 14, when they marched to Montmirail, stopping at Saint-Eugène overnight, a distance of about 29 miles.

On August 18, they traveled by truck from Saint-Eugène via Vitry, arriving at Liffol-le-Petit the next day, a distance of about 110 miles (map by author).

article in the Inquirer which said how much a home paper was appreciated over here. It only made one mistake. It said that the home paper was the most appreciated thing. They were wrong. The most appreciated thing is a letter. Sometimes we go a week or two without a letter. That is when it is hard to get any work out of the boys. When I opened the mail sack and took out the Sunday paper which you sent to me, it was almost as good as a letter. It had your hand writing on it and it had the personal touch. I saw that it was one that you had read and I looked in vain for places which you would mark out some article of interest which you would call my attention to. Of course the war news is read with great interest. It sure is great to read about something which takes up a couple of columns and say to yourself, I was there. You read tales and stories and you know about all of them and most of the time the interesting parts are taken out. Do you remember reading about how the second battle of the Marne was reported? Well I saw that news come back exactly as it was reported in the papers.

I said in the beginning of this letter we were going to move. I haven't the slightest idea as to where we are going but I suppose to some quiet sector. We have been wishing that we could be sent to Italy. We have certainly been blessed with good weather since we came over. It seems that most of the rain we have had has been at night.

I am enclosing a piece of the German airplane which was brought down in the battle. The machines are still out there where they fell. The aviators are still there too. The way they are buried is to kick a little dirt over them. One fellows foot is still sticking out of his grave.

Notice how this [the piece of the German airplane] is painted so as to make it invisible.

August 20, 1918

Tuesday

Liffol-le-Petit

We have moved to an entirely different front. Last Wednesday night [August 14] we marched from Chateau De La Foret to St. Eugene, France and arrived at 7:30 Thursday morning. Slept all day Thursday & Thursday night. Friday we marched from St. Eugene to Montmirail. On Sunday morning we loaded on trucks and traveled Sunday & Monday and arrived here. We passed thru a very beautiful country. We are in barracks now, this place is near Neuf Chateau. The country is quite mountainous here. The railroads are operated by American soldiers. [I] have been in a French town which has not been injured by the war. It sure is great.

Letter to family, August 23, 1918

I said in my last letter that we were moving. We left the last place and marched with full equipment. We marched all night thru part of the day. I lay down and slept the rest of the day and all night. Then we marched the next day and night. I found myself in a town so far behind the lines that it has not seen the destruction of war. It is French from top to bottom. There were lots of soldiers but the civilians were in place just the same.

Chapter 3. France

[A] quiet and quaint old French town. We left there and came across France in motor trucks. We did all of our traveling during the day. Therefore I was able to see quite a bit of the country.

I am in a rest area. It is far from the battle line. I am in a little old French farming town such as I have tried to describe to you before. When we came away from the lines, I had some strange feelings. When we left the line and came back to civilization little things which an ordinary mortal would not even notice came to my attention. I saw a railroad train and could smell the soft coal burning. No one had that alert look which is so noticeable at the front. The discipline was not so severe. It seems strange that the buildings were not shot down but were in perfect condition. There were no guns either during the day or night. One seldom sees an aeroplane and at night you don't have to sleep with your gas mask on. The town we are in now is about the size of Darby and of Collingdale when we first moved there.[22] There are no stores, and no doctors, no pharmacy. There are three saloons as we call them. Wine shops as they are known here. The American soldier is permitted to drink light wines and beer. This is in accordance with the general order from General Pershing. The soldiers are given much more freedom than in the States. Drunkenness is punished quite severely. Understand that men in the front never get a chance to buy booze so don't think Uncle Sam's boys go over the top drunk.

Good long letters are more appreciated than anything else. The Red Cross gave us each a package of tobacco. The donor's name was in each package. Mine was from someone named Harrington in Wilmington, Delaware.

Letter to family, September 5, 1918

I am glad you had a little trip for a vacation. I am sorry I was not with you but remember I am having a vacation too. I would not miss this for anything. We are still taking it easy. When the Division is up at the front there is little sickness. At least no one ever reports sick, but when you come back then up goes the sick rate. I saw Capt. McCall before he was buried.[23] I can't give you any details now. I may be able to remember them until I come home but there may be so many incidents that it will be impossible. I shall never forget the Second Battle of the Marne. I have hundreds of stories to tell about it—some funny and some serious.

Hospital working in a big drive is much different from what you would think. You read about beautiful females writing the last word to loving sweethearts. All bull! Take it from me. You read about the groans and the cries of the wounded and dying. I saw quite a few wounded and dying soldiers in that drive—American, French and German and I only heard three men make any noise. One was a Frenchman who was pretty badly shot up and the other two were Germans and they were more scared than hurt.

While the drive was at its height I passed through the shock ward. That is the ward where patients are taken after they have been operated on. This really is a ward for men too seriously wounded to be moved. There is not a sound except for a nurse talking to one of the boys. One fellow called me over and asked for a drink. I gave him some water. He asked me what time it was. I told and asked him where he was from: he said,

---

22. Darby and Collingdale are suburbs of Philadelphia.
23. Captain Howard Clifford McCall was the son of Joseph B. McCall, the president of the Philadelphia Electric Company. He was killed on July 26 while leading his battalion in battle.

"Altoona Pa." I asked him if he was hurt very badly, he said, "Well the Boche[24] are worse off than I am." I said, "How is that?" He answered, "Well, I got at least four of them and I don't know how many more." Here was his story:

He and another soldier and one officer were going thru a piece of wood. Just before they came to a ditch 6 Germans (an officer and 5 men) stood up and called Kammarade [Kamerad].[25] The officer detailed him to take them back. Just as they started the German officer turned and ran. The American shot the officer and then the German soldiers fired on the American. Well the Germans were all killed and the American boy was almost dead. He got as far as our hospital where a leg was cut off. About 10 minutes after he told me this, I passed through the room again. He saw me but his mind was wandering. He looked at me and said quietly, "Buddy, get one of those dirty suckers for me, will you? So long." And was that was his last words. No asking for home or letters or wishes or regrets.

The American boys come to France for just the reason that the Marines tell the Germans when they are captured (I guess the Germans don't capture very many) "To kill or be killed." And when a Yank does get it in the neck he doesn't cry over spilt milk. He just says, "Aw Hell, what's the difference."

I noticed your letter was dated August 6. Jerry came over and dropped a few shells last night as he did the night before. On the 5th of August he flew over us all night long. About 11 o'clock he dropped four pills in our front. Only three went off. He also woke me with another one about 3 o'clock in the morning.

I was in all the towns you mention (Vaux-Lorey). They are towns in name only. They resemble great big piles of brick and stone.

I met the officer to whom the credit of taking Vaux is given, He is a Second Lieutenant. "Shaved tail" is the Army name for a Second Lieutenant.

I can't realize that you're eating so called war bread. We have nothing like that over here. We eat straight wheat bread, all we want and always have some left over. Oh, I have eaten very hard tack and canned Willie too but not very often.[26] We feed so good that if you told anyone in the States how good it was you would be called a liar. We have moved again since I last wrote you and at present I am in a very famous part of France.

Letter to family, September 8, 1918,

As today was Sunday there were religious services held. I went this morning. I wish, oh I more than wish, that I can describe things that I see over here. I wish you could see soldiers at church. That is certainly an impressive service, far more impressive than a funeral service would be. To stand with it in a semi military service: The bugler blows "church call."

Today the service was held along side of a big ward tent. This tent is pitched on the side of the hill in the wood. Once in a while the silence is broken by the sound of a big

---

24. *Boche* was a French slang term for the Germans that apparently was originally derived from an old word for "head" that came to mean obstinate, stubborn, or pigheaded.

25. *Kamerad* in German means "Hey Buddy" or "Hey Pal." In this context, however, it meant "We surrender." It was sometimes used by the Germans as a dupe to make those to whom they were surrendering believe they were giving up by leading them into a deadly trap. Edward R. Coyle, *Ambulancing on the French Front* (New York: Britton Pub. Co., 1918), 141–50.

26. "Canned Willie"—sometimes called "Corned Willie"—was tinned corned beef that was detested by the soldiers.

Chapter 3. France

gun. When the church call was sounded the men who attended the service came and sat on the ground facing the ward tent. The service was conducted by a Y.M.C.A. man. He distributed small hymn books and a copy of the Psalms to each soldier. The "Y" man took his place near the tent and announced the first hymn. "Onward Christian Soldiers." There was no music, no harmony, no unison. Everybody just made a noise and we called it singing. But God doesn't care as long as your heart is in earnest—it matters little what the voice is saying or how it says it. Then we sang "Holy, Holy, Holy, Lord God Almighty."

The speaker was introduced. He did not take a text from the Bible but instead he took a Civil War story as his text and drew a lesson from that. He told how the Northern troops took Missionary Ridge. He only talked about 15 minutes. Then we sang again. Then a prayer and that was all.

Before the service started I looked the bunch over officers and men from Major down to buck privates. Hospital corps, Q.M. Corps, Engineers, Doughboys, from the Infantry, Artillery, Machine gun men and calvary. All arms and branches of service. Recruits and old soldiers, men who have been under fire and men who have not. Men who have killed other men in battle and men who have not. Hard looking characters and men from good families. Protestant and Catholic all sitting in that cosmopolitan crowd. Soldiers who have been through the fire and [have] been tried don't say much as a rule. They have that far away look. The trench face it is called. I would have called it the longing face—longing to have it over with and get back to God's country again. A soldier lives for today alone. There is no telling what tomorrow will bring or tonight as far as that is concerned.

After church I worked a little and then beat it to bed and took a nap. Not much to do this afternoon so I went out and walked for about two hours. That is how I get most of my exercise.

I am sleeping in my pup tent. It is surprising how comfortable the pup tent can be. I have plenty of blankets and I have no trouble keeping warm. The American papers are sure a source of pleasure to me. I read several incidents which I know to be true. Oh, I wish I could write and tell you of all the beautiful towns and cities I have seen and been thru and tell you of [the] destroyed towns. I mean their names. I have been to and thru many towns which were named in the papers during the end of July.

I have a box almost as large as a trunk in which I carry all my personal belongings. As the weather here in the summer is not as hot as in the states, I suppose that the winters are cold in proportion so I am preparing. I have a brand new suit which I have never worn. I have two pairs of knitted socks like grandmother made me. I have a sweater which I secured since mine was stolen and I have three suits of underwear and a new pair of shoes. I have no overcoat yet and I don't want to be bothered with one until winter. I need a helmet (knitted) but don't send any because the Red Cross will keep us supplied. The K of C (first), The Red Cross (second) and the Y.M.C.A. more than take care of us. The K.C. & R.C. things are free. The Y.M.C.A. charge.

Speaking of overcoats reminds me of the French soldiers. They are a mystery to the Americans. When our infantry march they carry their guns, their gas mask, their ammunition belt, their pack with their belongings and their canteen of water. Not so with the French. You see them in heavy marching order going into battle dress with their everlasting overcoat. They seem to never take it off. It makes no difference how hot it gets. That overcoat stays on. Then they have their rifle, their gas mask and their canteen filled with wine. It always been a mystery to me to find out where they carry their ammunition. You often see a French soldier swap his wine for American tobacco.

American soldiers are permitted to drink wine or beer but drunkenness is severely punished. Gen. Pershing is a very liberal with the men and permits much more personal freedom than soldiers are allowed in the states.

It is 9:30 PM here and a miserable rainy night. It is only about 3 or 4 o'clock in the afternoon with you and I suppose one of those delightful autumn afternoons. Perhaps this time next year I will be home enjoying it with you. Over here you never hear a soldier speak of the bad weather [that] we sometimes have in the states. To hear them talk you would think it was glorious springtime all the time.

Wednesday September 11, 1918

Vavincourt, France

Dear diary:—today is Julian's birthday.[27]

We arrived here about a week ago. We are about 15 miles from St. Mihel [Mihiel] and about 35 miles from Verdun. Passed through St. Dizier, and Bar-le-Duc. We crossed the place where the Rhine River starts. Bar-le-Duc is the largest town we have come to since we have been here. This front is very quiet. You seldom hear a gun fire. We are going to move up close to Verdun. We expected to go to Haudainville last week but it has been raining so hard lately we can't get out of this place. Things are certainly in awful shape.

Monday, September 9 was a Red letter day for me. I received my first letter from Marian. Not the first she had written but the first I received.

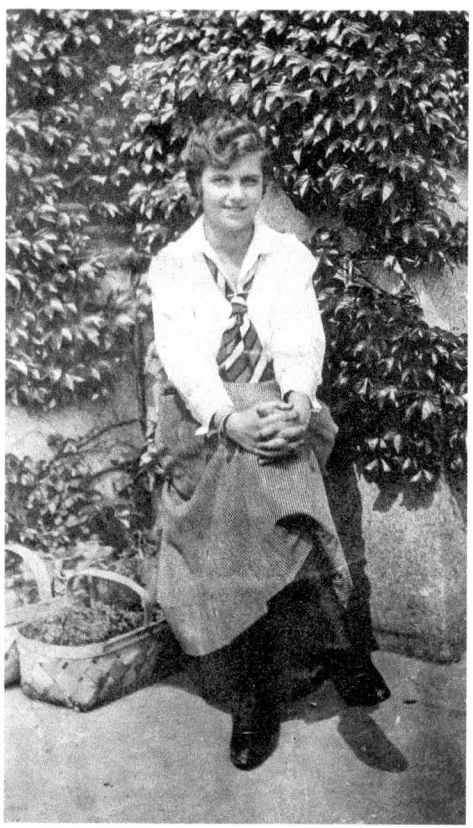

A photograph of Sergeant Brown's girlfriend, Marian, from his photo album. The first letter from her arrived on September 11—108 days from when he sailed from New York (photo album).

---

27. Julian Cotton Brown, a much-loved brother of Sergeant Brown, was born on September 11, 1896, and died on February 27, 1901, from diphtheria.

Chapter 3. France

Friday, September 13, 1918

Rambluzin, France

Arrived at this place to help the Corps Gas Hospital. We arrived in the rain and it rained ever since.

Editor's Note: Field Hospital No. 33 During the Saint-Mihiel Operation

From September 12 to 16, the 4th Division, of which Field Hospital No. 33 was a part, participated in the Saint-Mihiel offensive.

The Allied goal was to obtain the railroad center in Metz, which was an important supply center for the Germans, and to collapse the salient (bulge) held by the Germans since the beginning of the war. The weather did not cooperate: it rained for five days, making the roads almost impassable and the fields deep in mud.

On September 8, the Germans had withdrawn from the Saint-Mihiel salient to concentrate their forces east near the Hindenburg Line. The Saint-Mihiel offensive began September 12 with the 1st Corps on the right. Included within the 1st Corps was the 4th Division, Field Hospital No. 33 included.

The heavy use of air support by the Allies was evident. Almost 1,500 aircraft of 28 American squadrons were augmented by those of the British, French, and Italians. Together they constituted the largest air operation of the war. The American army was further aided by 110,000 French troops, which were also under General Pershing's command.

Tanks, which played a vital support to the infantry, were under American command of Lieutenant Colonel George Patton. As a result of careful planning and the depleted condition of the German army, the assault into the salient by the Allies was nearly unopposed. On September 12, the battle's first day, the objective was accomplished before noon, and by the afternoon of September 13, their second-day objective had been realized. General Pershing, seeing that the progress was going so well, ordered a quickening of the offensive. On the morning of September 13, all objectives had been met. Pershing ordered no further advances be attempted in order to prepare for the final offensive of the war: the Meuse-Argonne offensive.

Air support was led by Colonel "Billy" Mitchell. After the war, Mitchell was court-martialed and stripped of his rank because, among other reasons, he advocated the use of aircraft carriers over battleships. During this battle, Patton was severely wounded by a machine gun bullet. He would be remembered for his brilliant command of the tank corps in World War II.

In 36 hours on the battlefield, the Americans took more than 13,000 prisoners and captured 466 guns. The Germans lost 5,000 killed and wounded, while the Americans suffered 7,000 killed, wounded, or captured.

It is interesting to note that at the beginning of the Saint-Mihiel offensive, American soldiers who were bandsmen were previously prohibited to be used as litter-bearers. However, possibly because there was an expected need for additional litter-bearers in the Saint-Mihiel offensive, bandsmen were detailed from machine gun, rifle, supply, and headquarters companies to be used in this capacity. This arrangement provided 145 additional litter-bearers to be available as needed.

The 4th Division's Sanitary Train advanced to Haudainville and made Field Hospital No. 28 available for all classes of patients while Field Hospital No. 33 (Sergeant Brown's company) moved to Rambluzin to augment the gas hospital there. On September 19, they moved to Lemmes and on the next day to Sivry-la-Perche. From the records of the Army Medical Department, 522 patients passed through the triage of Field Hospital No. 28 while it was at Haudainville. While the Sanitary Train was at Lemmes, Field Hospital No. 21 received sick patients

Letter to family, September 13, 1918

Have been pretty busy for the past three days. I intended to write on September 11 (Julian's birthday) but on that day we moved. Rained all day. We were located in the wood and had to build a road thru the mud before we could get out. We broke camp and were out in the rain all day. It took us until dark to get loaded and out on the road. Then it started to rain harder and it got cold. I tell you it was no joke riding on top of those trucks.

We arrived at our new station at about 2 AM the next morning. Then we had to unload in the rain and mud. I met the first Sergeant of an ambulance co. which was here and he took me into his office. He turned on an electric light. I don't think anything surprised me as much as that did.

Well I took my blankets and made my bed on the floor. Then I took off my coat, my shoes and my leggings, rolled up on the floor and went to sleep. I slept until 8:30 in the morning. When I got up I pitched my big tent and fixed up my office.

I am sleeping in the office now. It is quite a cosy place [compared] to what we have been having. I have a cot now and I am trying to get a stove for the tent. If I succeed I will be at home again. I had to pitch a wet tent on wet ground and it has done nothing but rain since we arrived so you can imagine the circumstances.

I am in quite a famous part of the country.[28] It is beautiful around here. Of course the rain has helped to make it worse but I have been on top of a high hill. The country is hilly all around and is covered with trees. A French soldier told me that there were large deposits of coal and iron in this section.

---

28. He states that he is in a "famous part of the country." Perhaps famous as far as the war is concerned as he is near Verdun and Saint-Mihiel.

Chapter 3. France 81

Despite the poor weather there are more airplanes on this front than any other place I have been so far. Allied airplanes are coming and going all the time. Sometimes alone, sometimes in twos and threes and sometimes in squadrons. It's certainly pretty to see a large squadron of 20 or 30 planes (big bombers) flying in formation. I have come to the conclusion that airplanes are as safe as trans-atlantic liners. It seems that there are no accidents. The only men to get it are the ones killed in battle.

Well by the time you receive this letter I will have been in the army over a year. Sometimes I think it has been a short year and sometimes I think it has been a long year. There is one thing—I have certainly gained a bunch of experiences and I sure have seen things and had experiences and been to places that I would have not been to for perhaps years to come.

I think that I have gained quite a lot of self-assurance since I came in the army. I know that I have lost all timidity. I believe that I would have the guts to walk up to the King of England and say hello George, how's chances on a job? I[f] there's anything I want I walk up to anyone that it concerns and ask them about it. It makes no difference whether it is a private or a Colonel.—If I don't get it, well I don't and that is all. At least it means you are nothing out.

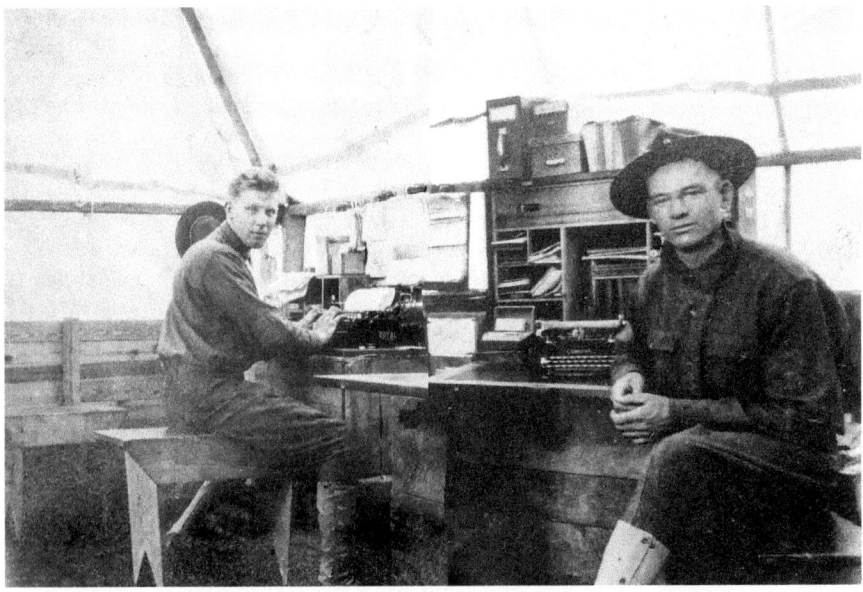

Two images of soldiers of Field Hospital No. 33 that are combined to make a view of Brown's office while in the field (photo album).

Letter to family, September 15, 1918

There are big doings here now. Sorry but I can't tell you about them. You are perhaps reading about them in the paper and know more than I do about the thing as a whole but I tell you it is sure great to be here. I want to tell you a few things about some of the towns that I have had the good luck to see. The first place that I got to know well was Meaux. I had to go through there a good many times and I always had plenty of time. I used to wander through the streets and alleys and its big cathedral. That place sure was a work of art from top to bottom. The streets are narrow and crooked and their shape reminds me of the streets and parts of Kensington near Richmond.[29] This town was a place where the Germans came nearest to Paris in their drive in 1914.

There were not very many German soldiers in the town [then]. The only ones which reached here were patrols. It was in this town that Marshall Joffer started the first Battle of the Marne. This river runs on, or rather, through the town. It is a small stream and not much wider than Darby Creek at Norwood.[30] It is very deep and the sides are very high. The banks do not run down gradually as do our rivers but you come to the edge of the bank and it falls abruptly down about 6 feet to the surface of the river and then down a depth of about 10 or 15 feet.

I went into a French Y.M.C.A. one day to get some coffee and cakes. I had an interpreter with me. We walked up to the counter where a woman was waiting on the Frenchmen. My friend and I were the only Americans in the place. He asked for our eats and then asked how we could get to another town we wanted to go to. She then spoke in English, "Suppose we talk English because I am an American." You have no idea how good it sounded to hear an American woman talk United States again.

The streets in the town (it is almost big enough to be called a city) are just as narrow as is possible to make them. The sidewalks are in front of some houses and not in front of others. No one ever walks on the sidewalks. We all use the street.

I was in this town about 2 months ago when the Boche were putting a long-range shell into the town every ten minutes. We could hear the shell coming long before it struck and we would bet which side of the town it would strike. It is surprising how exactly you can tell just which side of you the shells are going to land.

Meaux presents quite a contrast to Chateau Thierry. This is a town about the size of Meaux but when I was there it sure was one wrecked place. The streets of been cleared of all wreckage, but gee, you should have seen the houses. I don't believe there was a whole place in the town. I rode down the main street to a street which runs along the Marne River like Delaware Ave. along the Delaware River.[31] Just across the river was a place which manufactured wine. There was only about 3 holes in the building.

It was at Chateau Thierry that I first saw the German pillboxes. I stood on a hill near Vaux that looks down on Chateau Thierry. The town was spread out like a map. The only destruction which you could see was a blown up railroad bridge. Chateau Thierry lies in the most beautiful valley you ever saw. On the hills on the north side of the city were the pill boxes. It surely is a pretty part of France.

One afternoon while out for a walk I passed through the town of Lorey and was quite surprised to notice that the buildings were not so badly wrecked as in most places. Why this was I do not know. I went into Neuf Chateau one day. It is the largest city that I have seen over here. Believe me you can make yourself feel right at home.

One time I got to see the town of Vitry le Francoise. I was there on Sunday. In the center of the city was a big square just covered with people who were taking in a small traveling show that had pulled up there. There was a big cathedral on one side of the square and I think every other house on the square was a wine shop. I went into one

---

29. Richmond and Kensington are neighborhoods in Philadelphia near where he and his family used to live.
30. Norwood is a suburb southwest of Philadelphia.
31. Delaware Avenue in Philadelphia has been renamed Columbus Boulevard.

Chapter 3. France

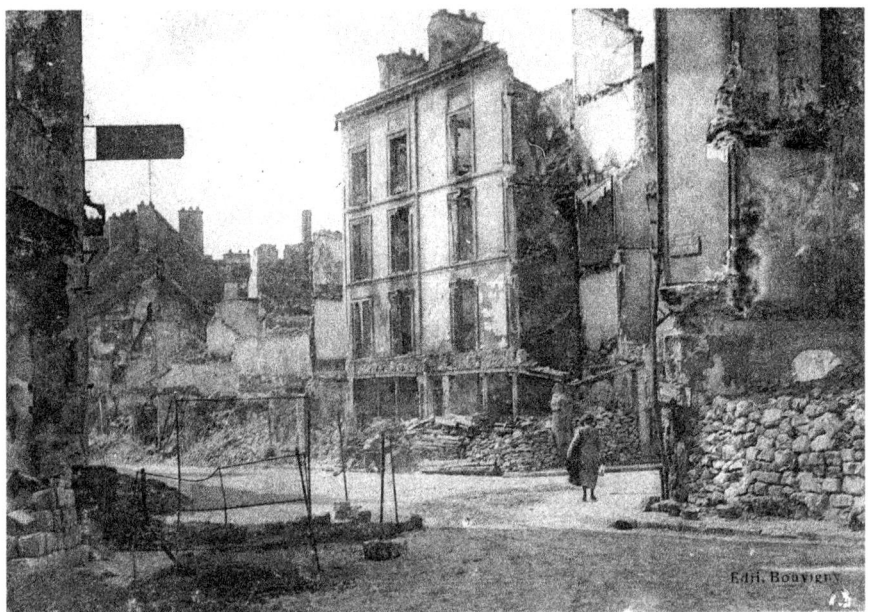

Postcard showing Château-Thierry, 1918 (Will Brown Collection).

and bought five boiled eggs and some fresh rolls. I don't remember when anything tasted so good. I was traveling by myself and had not stopped for much eating.

Just wait—I am going to see more of this country before long unless we move up into Germany. I wish we would be sent down into the sector Switzerland. I sure would like to see that country. I bet that it is pretty. I have talked to troops that have been down there and they all say that it is the prettiest place that they have ever been in. I hope that Germany is a pretty place because I know if it is not I will get homesick when we get there.

Thursday, September 19, 1918

Rambluzin, France

We are still on duty at this place. We have not done very much. We have been transferred to the 5th Army Corps. Gen. Cameron, our old division commander is C.O. of the 5th Corps. The 4th Div. was in the 2nd Corps then in the 1st [Corps] and at the request of General [?]

Friday Sept. 20, 1918

Lemmes, France

Last night we ate supper and prepared for bed. At 8 o'clock we received orders to move. The trucks arrived at 10 PM and the company left and marched to Lemmes. We arrived at about 4 o'clock this morning. We had to go into a woods. It was the thickest woods I have ever seen. We

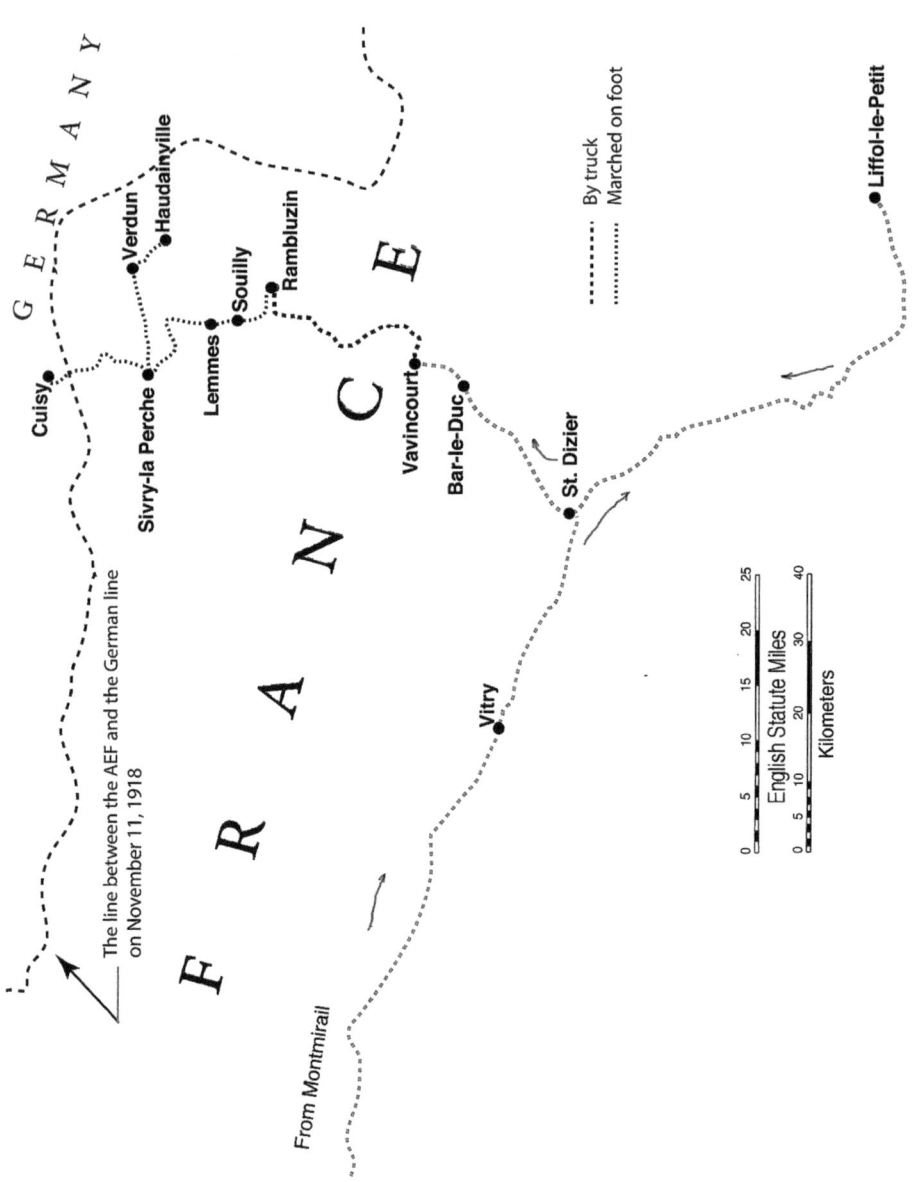

had to cut paths thru. Then we pitched our tents and went to bed. I hung the sign on my tent: "Quarantined, Leprosy. Keep out." That must have worked because no one disturbed me.

Saturday. September 21, 1918

Sivry [Sivry-la-Perche], France

Orders came at 10 this morning for us to move. We made the first daylight move that we had done since we arrived in France. We moved up to this place. It is about 7 miles from the line about four miles from Verdun and is in a little pocket. There are hills surrounding us. A good many of the houses in the place had been shot up. I have been assigned to a place which contains about 10 beds, double deck affairs. I am to have my office in here.

September 22, 1918. Sunday

Sivry [Sivry-la-Perche], France

Last night and today have been some day and night. I went to bed. I slept in my office. I had been asleep two hours when something woke me up. Then I heard what I thought was anti-aircraft barrage. Then silence. Then I heard report of a gun in the distance, then a whistle and then an explosion in the town. Then another explosion close by and then a shell hit my roof and fell alongside. It was a dud and did not go off but it knocked some of the shingles off the roof. It took me about six seconds to get my shoes and to reach the door. I stood there a few seconds and what I saw, sure was funny. Now I was scared but when I saw men scampering like rats I has [*sic*] sure did smile. But I beat it for a dug-out. I made that 100 yards in nothing flat. I passed about a dozen and they weren't standing still.

Now here's one on me. When I was standing in the dugout[32] (no light) I heard Sgt. Fisher and Rubley talking.

Fisher said, "Gee but didn't old Brown beat it quick?"

Rubley said, "He sure did. He must have been scared of them."

And I heard another voice close by say, "Well if there is anybody in

---

Opposite: **Vitry to Cuisy. On August 15, after the Aisne-Marne Offensive, Sergeant Brown, along with the 4th Division, traveled by truck from Château de le Fôret to Liffol-le-Petit, passing through Saint-Eugène and Montmirail and arriving on at Liffol-le-Petit on August 19, 1918. They were there for a period of rest, reorganization, and training.**

From September 4 to 12, his company moved to Rambluzin. On September 19, they marched to Lemmes, where they stayed overnight before moving to Sivry-la-Perche. On September 29, they relocated to Cuisy. He was gassed at Cuisy on September 30.

From Cuisy he was sent to the Evacuation Hospital No. 6 at Souilly on October 2. The following day he went by hospital train to Base Hospital No. 50 at Mesves. Mesves is southwest of Paris and is not shown on this map (map by author).

---

32. There was no particular dugout. It was usually a hole in the side of a hill that acted as protection against artillery fire.

here who is not afraid of them he had better move outside because he is taking up valuable room."

Believe me they piped down after that. Well I stayed in that dug-out for about two hours. Then I went back to my quarters again. Jerry had not sent out any over for about an hour. Just as I got into bed he started shooting again. I lit for that dug-out and stayed there until 5 o'clock. He kept shelling all the time. As I left my billet the second time a house next to mine was moved out into the street. He sure must have had my number written down.

He did not shoot anymore until 11 o'clock when he laid down three in succession along side of the kitchen. That was all he put over all day. It rained all day and that might have been the reason. About one quarter of the shells he sent over were duds. Reports come from troops from all the fronts that his ammunition is poor. Tonight I am going to sleep in the dug-out. I will be sure to get some rest. We are expecting an American drive. It may start any place from Reims to Verdun. My division has been handed the American or Allied right flank at Verdun. It is the hardest place on the whole line. Whatever this division has started out to do it generally finishes.

There is a castle on the German side of the line here-it is all reinforced and is really a fort. It is on a hill 342 feet high. As soon as it is captured then we will have nothing but a rolling unprotected country. At least that is the stories they tell.

Noman's land at this point is 3 miles wide. The Allies have [a] listening post a mile out. We are expecting a drive at any minute now. We are a Triage. All the other field hospitals have special duties. 28-Gas Hospital, 21-Divisional Sick and 19-Seriously Wounded. It is still cloudy and perhaps that is the reason why Jerry is not shelling us.

Sgt. Fisher has been recommended for Sgt. first class. He is to take the examination today or tomorrow.

Monday 23, Sept, 1918

Sivry-la-Perche

I slept in a dug out up on the hill last night. There was no shelling at all. I went to bed early and someone came in and woke me up. I told them to pipe down. Then he wanted a guard to watch for gas. I told him what a fool he was, that gas shells never came back that far. This morning when I woke up I found that the guys that I was telling to pipe down were officers. The Boshe only put three shells in this town today. They all came at 11 o'clock this morning. The 77th F.A. went into position on this front last night.[33] The artillery is moving up on this road now.

---

33. "F.A." means field artillery.

Tuesday September 24, 1918

I slept in a dug out with Idzikowski last night. The 16th F.A. Moved up last night. The German shelled the road on both sides of the town all night but I had a good night's sleep just the same. We received our first patients today. Towns have been shelled on both sides of us today. It has rained for two days and there sure is plenty of mud.

My shoes are wet and have been since it started to rain.

[Beginning of Volume 2]

Wednesday, September 25, 1918

Sivry-la-Perche, France

I have often thought of my grandmother's brother, who fought in the Civil War.[34] I remember very plainly of the thrills I had when I read the diary which he kept in 1863. I remember how I used to wish that he would have been more fuller in his explanations of his experiences. I hope that I may write a full story of my part over here so that I may refresh my memory as soon as I get home.

Well last night I decided to sleep in my billet instead of going over to a dug out. I slept here instead. About 4 o'clock this morning an American battery about a kilometer from here opened up. It sure did have a funny effect on me. I lay in bed and shook, just as if I had malaria but I went to sleep soon and did not hear any more until reveille this morning. Yesterday was fairly clear and there was lots of activity in the air. The German observation planes were over our lines for quite a while and did not seem to mind our aircraft barrage.

Today has been cloudy and fairly cool and we have a fire. The first one I have been near in France.

Here is the picture of a girl that Sgt. Bowman and I write to. I will write the letter and Bowman dictates it.

This morning there was an Allied ascension or observation balloon put up on the other side of the hill from where we are. It is the sausage shaped type. It wasn't up 15 minutes before it was hauled in. Then the anti-aircraft went to work and we saw a German plane. Finally a shrapnel shell

---

34. His grandmother's brother was William Fletcher Nelson, who was born in 1842 and died on June 18, 1864, near Petersburg, Virginia, as a result of Confederate attack.

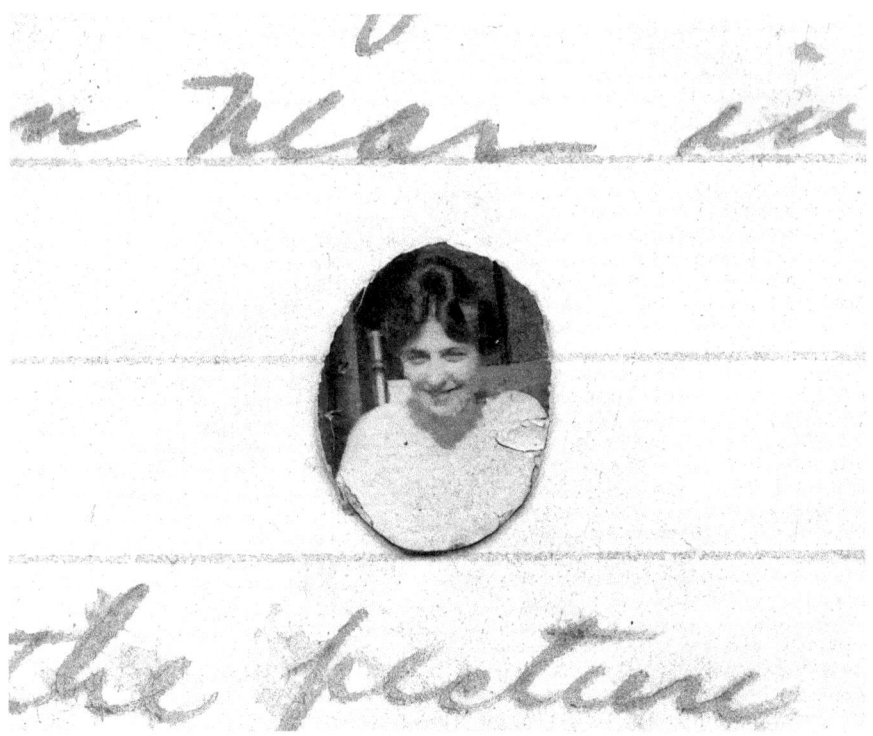

In his letter of September 25, 1918, from Sivry-la-Perche, France, Leland speaks of writing letters to this young woman with Sergeant Bowman. He included this photograph with that letter (photo album).

exploded near the plane and it came down in flames. Right after this the balloon was put up again. Then hauled in again and I saw six Jerries trying to pass the lines again but the barrage was so thick they had to go back.

Things are quiet as far as artillery is concerned. There have been no German shells back here so far today and the heavy artillery located near us has only put over about a dozen shells all day.

Editor's Note: The Meuse Argonne Offensive, September 26–November 1, 1918

After their success in the Saint-Mihiel operation, the Allied forces planned to continue to push the German army further to the east, with what has become known as the Meuse-Argonne offensive. This began on September 26, 1918, and lasted until the Armistice on November 11, 1918, a total of 47 days.

The German supply railroads ran parallel to the front and

were essential to the German war effort. With the convergence of the three major armies—the French, the British, and the American—against the Germans on the Western Front, the Allies hoped to gain control of the railroads. In some areas these were within 10 miles from the front. They were well defended, with extensive lines of barbed wire, trenches, and other fortifications that extended about 10 miles or more behind the front lines. The Meuse River gave the Germans an advantageous natural water obstacle. Also, the Germans controlled the high ground, another advantage over the Allied armies.

The Allies' plan was to divide the German army toward different sides of the dense Argonne Forest, disrupting their supplies. The American army, with the French on its left flank, would advance toward Metz. The British troops would advance toward Saint-Quentin and Cambrai.

The operation was one of a series of Allied attacks that brought the war to an end. The addition in France of 1,200,000 American ground troops to augment those of the French, British, and Belgians had clearly altered the balance. Yet it took 47 days of difficult fighting, with many causalities, to bring Germans to an unconditional surrender. This was a far more difficult battle than those in Saint-Mihiel.

The battle cost Germany 120,250 causalities (28,000 killed and 85,786 wounded). American causalities were 122,063 (26,277 killed and 95,786 wounded).

It was the largest battle in United States military history.

September 25, 1918, 8:15 PM

Tonight is supposed to be the night of nights. There has not been much activity tonight. There was an aeroplane which came over. It flew above the road here and dropped a tube.

The hill behind which we are stationed is the place from where the Army officials are going to watch the battle. Everything is ready. On my sector there are over 200 14 inch guns. The light field artillery is up hub to hub deep. The infantry is in position, Machine guns are in place. We are only awaiting the word. The front to be attacked is said to be over 100 km in length. 300,000 French and 300,000 Americans are to be placed in the line. The situation of the British front is this. They have reached St. Quentin. It was quite a nut to crack last year. It is part of the Hindenburg Line. If Germany is weakened at some other place she might have to move some troops from St. Quentin. An attack at Verdun might mean that the Allies could flank St. Quentin from the Germany left. That's the way it looks to me. A Master Signal Sergeant told me that the Germans were replacing the troops who held this sector with Austrians. That means first that they have some kind of information as to this movement and second that our job will be a little bit easier.[35]

It is three minutes to nine. There is not the sound of one gun. We are all ready. Everything is in place. The ambulances are at the front. Military police are up and ready to receive prisoners. The prisoner pens near the railroad are empty and guards are on duty. Everyone is walking around restlessly and talking in whispers. This means that we are waiting for the zero hour.

September 26, 1918, 1:27 AM Thursday

The offensive is on. About 9:30 last night I was called out to see a light which was floating from the German lines. It was cloudy. Not a dozen stars were to be seen. This light was about the size of a star. It came down [and] passed over our heads and went on. Shortly after this the Germans started shelling the road on either side of the town. He was putting a shell over about every five minutes. Our batteries were absolutely silent. Ammunition trucks were passing up to the front over [the] shelled road. And the sky cleared off. I sat in the receiving ward. Cases were coming in pretty fast. They were the usual bunch who always came up to the hospital before a battle. Most of them complained of cramps or else they were shot in the arm or leg. Just such cases as you always doubt as to their being genuine. It looked more like malingering but we gave them the benefit of the doubt. About 11:30 another of the floating lights appeared. These lights mean that the enemy is trying to see if the wind is right for gas. We watched this light for quite sometime.

Exactly 11:40 a signal rocket flared up directly in front of us. I wish I could record the results with motion picture and photograph. The sky lighted from the N.W. to the Southeast. The roar was terrible. Then hundreds of signal rockets. Then the big heavy artillery resumed firing just as fast as they could load. Every time a big gun would fire one or more flashes would be sent off some distance away from the gun. The object of this was to make it hard for the enemy to locate the positions of the gun flash. They had one guess in three. Down toward Verdun, the enemy replied to this fire with shrapnel. I could see it burst in the air. Exactly at 12 o'clock all the light artillery opened up by firing one round. Every gun fired at the same

---

35. The Meuse-Argonne offensive, also known as the Battle of the Argonne Forest, was a major part of the final Allied offensive of World War I that stretched along the entire Western Front. It was fought from September 26, 1918, until the Armistice of November 11, 1918, a total of 47 days. The Meuse-Argonne offensive was the largest in United States military history, involving 1.2 million American soldiers, and was one of a series of Allied attacks known as the Hundred Days Offensive, which brought the war to an end. The battle cost 28,000 German lives and 26,277 American lives.

time. The enemy stopped shelling the road until about 1 AM and they have occasionally put one over since that time. Every half hour the light artillery fires one round. Every gun speaks at the same time. There is a battery on the other side of the hill from me. It sure does shake the place. So far, neither side has sent out any aeroplanes.

When Germany started out in 1914, she wanted a military decision. I feel quite sure that she is going to get it. I don't think that she is going to be satisfied even then. At 2 AM I understand that there is to be another kind of a barrage start[ing]. It is 1:55 AM now. I am going to wait to see what happens. Then I shall go to bed.

5:04 AM 26 September 1918

Well I didn't go to bed at 2 o'clock as I said I was going to do. We had an American officer brought in wounded. He said that we were attacking on a front of 127 kilometers. I sat and talked to one of the men, Shimska [Schimska], for a little while and then I crawled into a cot and just as I dozed off, the barrage increased in fury. Then I went out and watched it for a little while and finally Sgt. Hodsdon and I went up on top of the hill (Hill 347 I think is its number). We could see the country from 25 kilometers east of Verdun to 35 kilometers west. What we really watched it from were the trenches with which the French defended Verdun against the Germans attack in 1915. I could see the Allied Guns for miles around. First I would see the flash, then I would hear the shell fall and finally I would hear the report from the gun.

I saw an enemy ammunition dump go skyward. It certainly was a beautiful sight. The first thing I noticed was a ball of fire which looked like the great, big, yellow, harvest moon. This drew larger and larger and finally a spurt of flame came out of the top like a volcano. Then it died down. A full two minutes later the hill shook with two tremendous explosions.[36]

Hodsdon and I watched the scene for about an hour and a half.

Walters is talking in his sleep. He said, "Well we are laying down a sidewalk to Berlin."

September 26, 1918, 3:30 P.M.-

Went to bed at 5:30 this morning. Woke up at 7:30. Ate some breakfast, made out some reports and went to bed again. I slept in Sgt. Bowman's billet. I think I am lousy again. I was awakened about 11:30 by a big naval gun which was mounted on a truck. It pulled up on the road just behind my billet. I thought that the place was coming down. I got up,

---

36. If it took two minutes for the sound of the explosion to reach him, he would have been about 25 miles (40 kilometers) from it.

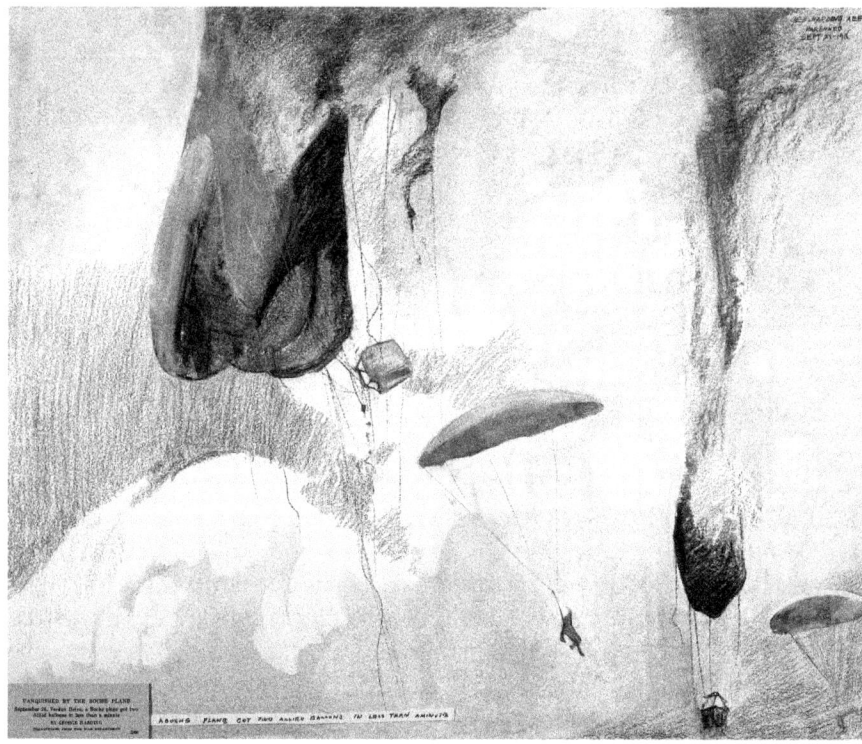

"Vanquished by the Boche Plane." The caption reads: "September 26, Verdun Drive, a Boche plane got two Allied Balloons in less than a minute." This watercolor by George Harding, a war artist for the U.S. Army, shows the same downing of the observation balloons as described by Sergeant Brown (Division of Political and Military History, National Museum of American History, Smithsonian Institution).

dressed and went to the company [mess] and ate dinner. Then I went to work in the receiving room. The barrage had died down and there was not much noise. This morning bright and early our observation balloons were out. They were protected by aeroplanes but this afternoon they were no aeroplanes. About 2 o'clock a German aeroplane dropped out of the sky. Shot his machine gun a couple [of times] and two of our observation balloons came down. An Allied plane came along and chased the Boshe. We had the pleasure of seeing him brought down.

Now about the reports which we are receiving. We hear that the Americans have advanced 8 km. They reached their objectives. We heard that 17,000 [German] men have been captured including one general and three truckloads of officers. We have handled about 200 wounded. That is a good many to come in broad daylight. About 40 of them were

Germans. Two were officers. I am going to try—(Get the try) to get some sleep tonight.

Evening September 27, 1918

I slept like a rock last night. We continue to receive wounded from the front. Field Hospitals 21 and 19 moved out. They moved up to Cuisy. F.H. 28 is still running a Gas Hospital with us.

We received a copy of the New York Herald which says that our men were advancing. There's been quite a lot of heavy artillery today. I think that this front is harder than they thought it was. I feel sick tonight. I am going to go to bed early.

Letter to family, September 28, 1918

This makes the third letter I started to write you since last Sunday. I try to write every Sunday at least. I did not write Sunday because the Boche shelled us all Saturday night and Sunday. We pulled into a town very close to the line on Saturday afternoon in broad daylight. Something which neither side seldom does. I was just tucked comfortably in bed when Bang! I thought the house was down. Then another shell burst. I started after my shoes and leggings when the third shell came over and knocked a hole in the sidewall and punctured a hole in the roof over my bed, filling my bed with stones and dirt. It landed in the backyard.

Wonders will never cease. It did not explode but believe me it was a close call. I got out of the house. Well the Boche shot for about two hours. Then I went back and as I was cleaning up my bed he put a shell in our front yard. Let me tell you I went out of that house and stayed out of the rest of the night. On Sunday he shot quite a bit, but most of the shells went in other parts of the town. I haven't decided which is worse—high explosive shells or aerial torpedoes.

Well the second time that I started to write I was interrupted by the offensive which started. I sat up all night to watch it. We knew when it was going to start. Have you ever been in an amateur theatrical? Do you know the breathless minute before the curtain rises? When this started it reminded me very much of that. Everything was ready in place. Our men at the hospital were in their places. The military police were ready to receive prisoners. The prison near the front was empty. The ambulances were at the front. The guards were on duty. The men were walking about restlessly and talking in whispers. It meant that we were waiting for the zero hour.

It was a beautiful night. The moon came out and threw everything into relief. I walked out of the office and joined some officers and noncoms who were standing in front of a ward tent. Between me and the line was a big hill. Suddenly I saw a single rocket. Before it reached its full height a roar such as I have never heard before broke out. The sky lighted from horizon to horizon. Then silence. Then the guns spoke at random. First here and then there, oh can't describe them. My mind works faster than my hand. I spent the rest of the night on the hill.

I saw a German ammunition dump blowup. It rose like a ball of fire just as a big yellow harvest moon would come up over a hill. Then the top broke and a spurt of flame came out. It took full two minutes for the sound to reach us. I even felt the concussion.

It must've been 20 km from where I stood. And now, well we don't know much about it. We do not get newspapers or news. Once in a while we hear artillery but not the big stuff. All small.

When I was in the Chateau Thierry sector, I wrote and told you that I saw Lieut. Quentin Roosevelt fall. I did not tell you but afterward I saw his grave. Quite a simple affair and just where he fell.[37]

Well I enlisted just one year ago today. Then I was in hundreds of miles from the line and scared to death. Now I am right up against it and it does not worry me in the least. That just shows the difference in our feelings.

For dinner today we had "slum." That is the army name for stew. I had about a quart and [I] have a small appetite. I do not want to write every time we are bombed or shelled. Every soldier has those experiences. Our work is very much varied. Sometimes we act as a sick hospital. It is then that we handle all the divisional sick. Then we act as a wounded hospital. Then we do all the work on [the] slightly wounded. Then we might act as a "triage." By that is meant that we sort out the sick and the wounded as they are sent to us from the line.

My work is just the same as it was in the states. I look out for the records. I have two separate departments—1st the hospital with patients and 2nd the company. I have two separate shifts. Now we are acting as a triage and a sick Hospital. My work is about double but I am getting away with it.

My work is overseeing. I do not do much work with my hands. I say yes or no or do it this way or that way. As to learning French I think I know less than I did before I came over. I talk to all the German prisoners that come in to get their records. At first I had quite a little trouble but now I get on fairly well with them. The German soldiers on the front are very young or else over age. They belong to the reserve divisions and not to combat divisions.

You ask how the war is going? Alright as far as I can see. I was in the St. Mihiel business but that was done so quickly and neatly that there was not much work for us to do.

I have two pairs of knitted socks the Red Cross gave me. I am holding onto them too, you can bet. There was quite a supply of them while the weather was warm, but no one wanted them then. I took two pairs and now most of the boys would like to have them. I have lugged them all over France and now I would not part with them for anything. I was sorry to lose the ones that grandmother made for me. I think that was the last thing she made for me.[38] *I have everything for my comfort except I wish I could get some ice cream and some chocolates. We get some sweet cakes and we are also able to get some sweet chocolate but I do not like it. The chocolate is granular like the penny pieces they sell the children. One of our boys received some candy from England ordered thru an American firm. He gave me some and it was just like we get at home and I sure did enjoy it. I have had nothing over here that tasted better.*

Oh yes I have cooties. I have been trying to get rid of them for about three weeks but am not very successful. Last week I was a small town. Today I was looking over the personal columns on my shirt to see if there were any new arrivals and I found that now I am a big city. It must be a convention by the way they are flocking in on me.

---

37. Quentin Roosevelt was the youngest (and favorite) son of President Theodore Roosevelt.

38. His grandmother who knitted the lost socks was his father's mother, Annie Nelson. She died in 1918, just before he shipped over.

Chapter 3. France 95

Letter to family, October 13, 1918

I have been pretty sick since I wrote you last. I have had influenza.[39] *I have not felt well for a month and on the first of this month I had to go to bed. They looked after me fine but I got worse so I was sent to the Base Hospital and here I am. Today is my first day out of bed and I sure am shaky. When I walk I wobble like a drunken man but I think I shall be O.K. in a couple of weeks. I hope so at any rate. I have been away from my outfit for almost two weeks. I have had no mail. There should be quite a bunch for me.*

This hospital is located in the very center of France and when I came down I rode in one of the U.S. Army Hospital trains. They sure are the greatest things I have ever been in. The beds are as comfortable as you would have in a first-class American Hotel. When I go back to my outfit I don't suppose I shall travel in such style.

This hospital is right in the center of grape country. White grapes and blue grapes. I bought some white grapes the other day and they are like white grapes we buy at home in the counter. But these are fresh. Gee but they were good. I bought two francs worth and got about 4 pounds. I wish you folks could have tasted them with me.

Today is Sunday and I have been wondering whether you had hotcakes and sausage for breakfast.

Letter to family, October 17, 1918

I am coming along fine. I sure feel much better. This trip to the hospital has been a vacation and a real rest. I believe it is the first time in the last five years that I have had absolutely nothing on my mind to worry about. Even my vacation while I was with Mr. Holland I worried about this and that and when I had my first furloughs [and] since I have been in the army there were things to worry about.[40] *But now I feel like a kid at the beginning of a vacation. I have lost quite a bit of weight, but I am coming along fine now.*

My goodness but how I do eat. I am ashamed of myself at every meal. The head nurse in our ward is giving me a little job. I am taking care of the temperature book for her. It gives me something to do. And something to help pass away the time. I have had no mail from you or anyone else since I have been here in the hospital. That is about three weeks now. It sure is hard to be with out news from home for all that time.

They are going to allow us to have a box from home for Christmas. It is pretty small in size (9 × 4 × 3). I don't suppose you will be able to get much in a box of that size.[41] *I don't know what I want you to send me. I suppose the newspapers at home will have suggestions. Don't send any knitted goods. The Red Cross supplies all of that. Oh how I*

---

39. Not wanting to worry his family that he was gassed, he told them that he had contracted influenza, probably not realizing that more soldiers were dying of influenza than in battle.

40. Harry B. Holland was Leland's preceptor in college. He became a partner in Holland's drugstore after the war.

41. The 3 × 4 × 9 was the size of the box that the family was allowed to send to their overseas soldier. The regulations: Only one package may be sent to each soldier. Christmas parcels must be placed in cardboard boxes 3 × 4 × 9 inches provided to holders of labels by the American Red Cross. They must not weigh more than two pounds and 15 ounces. Perishable food, soft candy, liquids, or anything in glass containers would be subject to removal. Parcels were to be taken to the nearest Red Cross collection station, where they would be inspected and then sent to Hoboken, New Jersey, from where they would be sent overseas.

wish I could have one of my chocolate cakes. I have craved some of mother's cakes ever since I have been in France. That is one thing I can't buy. I have trouble getting candy. The French don't have any candy like ours. They use a lot of chocolate but take it from me, it sure is cheap stuff. It is not at all like Hershey's but like the stuff we pay a penny for. I can get all of that I want but I do not like it.

We had some corn bread the other day. It was served hot. Oh gee, I never knew it was so good. We are so far from the line that we are allowed to send postals with the names of the towns on them.

This part of France sure is pretty. I had high hopes of peace but it looks like six more months of it. Never mind tho if we can't come home this Xmas we will be by the next one.

Germany can't last much longer. It sure is a shame that something doesn't happen to the Kaiser and bust the whole works.

Letter to family, October 20, 1918[42]

Well I am still in the hospital. I feel much better than I did a week ago when I wrote you last. I have sent to my outfit for my mail, but as yet, I have not heard from them. I suppose there will be a big batch up there for me. I hope so at any rate. It was quite hazy as to the date I went to bed. It was September 28th. I am still weak and nervous and I tire out quickly. I go for a little walk each day and I am always glad to get back to my bed. I think that I was completely rundown. I have not been feeling well since the first of September. I walked around in a sort of daze. I felt fine up until then.

All summer long we had the finest sunny days that anyone would want but for the past two months it seems to rain all the time. Today however is an exception. The sun is shining fine and I am sitting outside my ward taking it all in. The doctor and the nurses here sure are fine. They treat me Royal. They let me do a little work. It helps pass away the time.

I am still enjoying the grapes that grow in the district. They are bought up so fast that I can only get them about twice a week.

I have a sort of scrapbook in which I put newspaper clippings.

Letter to family, October 28, 1918

Yesterday was Sunday and it was such peach of a day that I went for a walk. I am coming along fine now. The town I went to was about four kilometers from the hospital. This town was the first French town that I have seen that had not been shot at or bombed. The town is built on both sides of the two streets that run into each other like a letter T.

There was not a new house the whole town. Most of the houses were built before the flood but there were one or two places which might have been built within the last hundred years. They sure were fancy affairs but too ginger Bready for us Americans.

There was a photographer in the town. He claims to have a special appointment as [the] photographer to the President of France.

There is a railroad near us. I often walk out to watch the trains. The locomotives interest me. The American government has quite a lot of engines and cars over here. It

---

42. September 20 was his birthday. He would have been 25 in 1918.

Chapter 3. France

sure does make us feel good to see them. The French locomotive is just as large as ours but they have a whistle that you would never recognize as a locomotive whistle. The French locomotive never has a bell on it. Our machines over here do. I see quite a number of privately owned automobiles back here. Gasoline for private use is $1.50 per gallon.

I am getting better all the time and I have had no mail since I came to the hospital.

Letter to family, November 10, 1918

Another week is gone by since I last wrote to you and I start this letter with the hopes that I can write 6 or 8 pages But way back here in the S.O.S. there is no more excitement than you find in Collingdale.[43] This week finds me better than last.

I have been doing work for an officer who has charge of several wards. My work for him has been satisfactory and I am to be more or less permanently attached to this hospital. Now that means that I cannot be transferred here permanently but they put me on detached service. My work here will last until sometime in the spring. Then it is up to him as to whether I shall stay or go back to my field hospital. At least I shall be sure of a good clean bed from now until then. I shall be sure of eating three square meals a day every day instead of taking a chance on chow like I used to do. And last and best I shall be out of the wet.

The seasons in France are all different from ours. The summer is beautiful. The fall—well it started to rain about the first of Sept. I believe it rained every day in that month. Then October came and perhaps I saw the sun on five days. In another month the snow starts and then the cold until it begins to rain again.

This morning I read a bunch of newspapers. There sure is a bundle of news in the home papers which we never get in the papers that we buy over here. We are very anxious to get news of the attack on Metz but that city is hardly mentioned in the papers. I read about it more in the papers you just sent me. Don't be afraid to mark anything you want to call my attention to. The authorities do not care if you do and besides anything published in American papers is all right.

I was sorry to learn of the death of Capt. Lynch but we see so much of suffering and see so many picked off that we have hardened ourselves to it.

News came this morning of the abdication of the Kaiser. There is a German prisoner of war sleeping in the bed next to mine. He was just as much tickled over the news as I was. Should the war [be over] and peace signed within the next 3 or 4 months, I do not think that I will be sent home for sometime. Gen. Pershing says that the first ones over will be the first ones home so you can see that puts me way down the list. Then I suppose the engineers and the medical men will stay to do reconstruction work.

Now as long as I am almost well I am going to tell you why I was sent to this hospital. I was gassed and almost had pneumonia. But remember I am almost alright now. I did not want to worry you about me. It sure is a great tale and I am one of the lucky ones who lived to tell the tale.

I am enclosing some pictures of the town located near the hospital. It is quite a thriving French city. The name of the town is La Charite. The river is the Loire and the department is Nievre. I want to see Paris and Nice and Aix-les Bains before I come back.

I have not been paid since August 31. I still have some money left. The two month

---

43. "S.O.S." refers to service of supply (see the glossary).

wages due me means that I have saved that much money. So I am going to have some money when I hit the states. I have had no more mail (letters) from you since I came to this outfit.

The papers this morning sure did make me feel good.

Letter to family, November 12, 1918

"Wal, wal, wal who would uv think it."

"The bloody blooming thing is over."

You know you hear rumors all the time. The old dame sure does hold full sway in the army. Of course we knew we were about to sign the armistice but nobody would believe it was really finished. Just let me tell you about a model conversation.

A fellas stepped up to another and said

"The guerre will be finée at 11 bells"

"Finée la guerre?"

"Bull! you're a liar"

"Yep, eleven o'clock"

"Ring off, that's old stuff, that rumor"

"Want to bet on it?"

"Who told you?"

"The Major says so."

"Hell, who is he? I'll wait until Genl. Foch comes an tells me himself."

And so it went and then we rec'd a copy of the Paris edition of the New York Herald. I am going to keep it as a souvenir. It said, "The war is won." We began to believe it then.

Well I am a veteran of the great European war. I have a service chevron and a wound chevron. I am glad that I enlisted. I am glad that I am with the Regulars. I would not be a bit surprised if my Division was sent to Germany to do police duty. I may be over here for a year more. I can now think of the future. I surely wish I was rolling pills again.[44]

Letter to family, November 15, 1918

The scrap is over. Perhaps we shall be on our way back in six months or a year. I should rather come back in the summer. Things are a lot better then. I came over as to a frolic. I found it a serious determined business. A trade which exacted the utmost of each of us. He who did not play the game right with the knowledge and preparedness paid the extreme penalty or suffered injury. I am glad that I served my country. I will be and I am now proud to say that I was there. I saw it. I experienced it. There is nothing which has pleased me more. I am proud of my service chevron and my wounded chevron.[45] It has been a wonderful experience. I hope the days will fly till I come back.

I read Alan's letter. Just think you wrote that more than two months ago and that night I was marching up a road to the front. It was raining. It was cold. It was dark. I could just barely see the back of the man in front of me. I started to march about 7:30. By 8 o'clock my feet and legs were soaked thru. Then the rain started down my back. At 3 o'clock in the morning I reached my destination. It was a wooden building and here

---

44. "Rolling pills" refers to his work as a pharmacist; he made pills by rolling the medicine into cylinders, which he then cut into small disks or pills, sometimes rolling these into little balls.

45. He never received a wounded chevron. It appears that if one was gassed, it did not count as being wounded.

was to be our hospital during a drive which sure has become famous. There was no way to change clothes so I had to roll up in my blanket and go to sleep. A few days after this the drive came off. It was a success. Then we waited here for a while. Then another night march. Slept in the daytime and march at night. At last we arrived at our destination. Then we were shelled for several days. I have already written you about that. Then a new drive started. I have also told you about that.

Several days after that drive started we were ordered up closer to the front. The town we were ordered into had not been cleared of Germans. I could see German snipers and machine gunners firing out of the windows, shell holes and trees. But the Yankees slowly but surely closed in on them. We set up our hospital. Everything went fine. Once in a while a shell would come over. Then came the gas. I got mine. Not much in the eyes or lungs but plenty on the body. Then I was out of the game. Now the war is over. I shall have a bunch of stories to tell you.

I sure do enjoy every paper I can lay my hands on. The clipping you sent me does not affect me at all. You say I was not in the S.O.S. but I was continually with the combat troops. [S.O.S. means Service of Supply, or service of the rear].

Letter to family, November 18, 1918

I received a letter today with the photographs of you all and Mr. and Mrs. Rooney. It was dated Oct. 10th. Your letters arrive in bunches. We get mail every day and when I do not get any I am disappointed. The photos which you sent me and the ones before are great. They make me feel that home is not so very far away. I wish that I can come home now and get some of that good "chow" which you write and tell me about. Oh! for some of that jelly.

Letter to family, November 24, 1918

Mesves, Bulcy, France

The lid is off. We can say what we please. We can mention towns. Yes, I was at Mihiel but we were up near Verdun. I have been through Verdun several times. I think there were only two cities in Europe that I really was anxious to see. One was Verdun and the other was Paris. I have seen Verdun, now for Paris. I was in the last big American offensive (the offensive which the American started near Verdun). I was at a town N.W. of Verdun called Sivry La Perche and then at a town which I have forgotten the name of. I think it was called Comey. It was up past the old German front line [the town was Cuisy].

The Germans have wonderful artillery and take it from me I have all the respect in the world for it. But the Americans are just as good, perhaps better. The god of war sure does some funny things and some of the customs over here are very amusing. Prisoners interest me. I like to talk to them. When the French captured a German the first thing they do is cut off all his buttons off the clothes. Then the prisoners can't run away without their trousers coming off. Americans are different. The prisoners are treated fine. They are put in tents near American hospitals. A "P.W." is painted on their clothing but there is no guard kept on them. They are allowed to go wherever they wish and they are not all dumb either.

The battle San Mihiel surely was a cleanup. My hospital had just one wounded man. Lots of sick but no one wounded. I am okay and I am not going to say anything more about my health unless I get sick again.

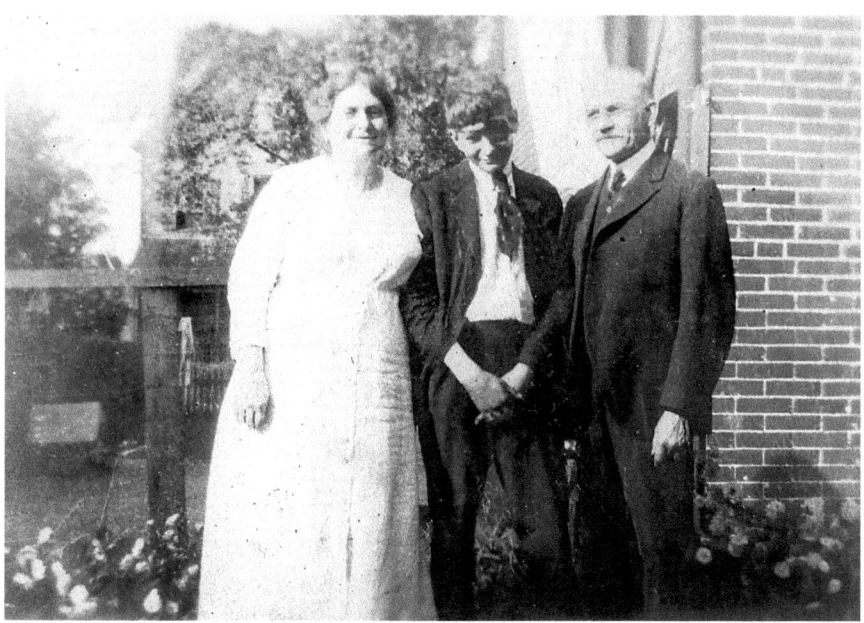

Leland's mother, Nora; his brother, Alan; and his father, Will, in their backyard in Collingdale, Pennsylvania (photo album).

Letter to family, November 30, 1918

It may be of interest to you to know that the place where my sweater and socks were stolen was at Meaux, France. It was the town where the French stopped the Germans in 1914. It was shelled quite often last summer although it was 50 miles from the line. I was there one day when it was being shelled. Did I ever tell you that I was at Chateau Thierry, St. Mihiel, Verdun, Rhiems [Reims], Soissons, Paris, Le Havre, Liverpool, England and Southampton?

I am a long way from home but I sure do wish that I was back in Philly with my feet under Mrs. Brown's table again.

Chapter 4

GASSED

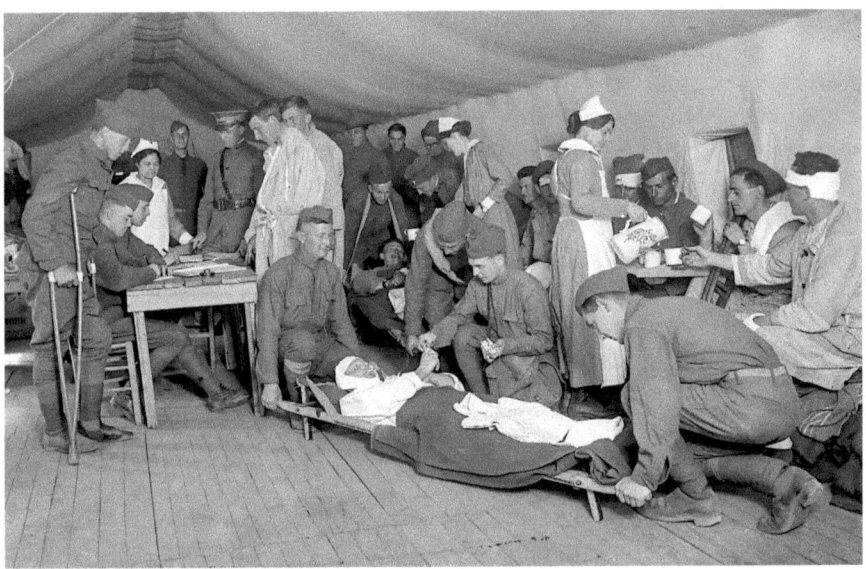

Receiving wounded at an evacuation hospital, photograph by Lewis Wickes Hines (Library of Congress).

Dec. 6, 1918 Base Hospital #50
Mesves-Bulcy, France
Well diary old man, it has been just two months and nine days since I had you in my hands. I have been writing on scraps of paper since I saw you last and now I am going to copy the whole story of the past two months. I will copy the dates as I wrote them on the papers.

Nov. 8, 1918
Mesves-Bulcy-France
On Sept 28, word reached us that the English in Flanders, the Belgians

in Belgium and the French on the rest of the front has opened up. An infantry officer came into the hospital and told us that we have been pushed back and that we were up against a stiff proposition. He outlined for us the military value of a drive on this front. If we are able to push the Germans back to Luxembourg, we will have cut all of their direct lines from Flanders to Lorraine and we also will be able to outflank the town of Metz.

I am sort of hazy about the dates but I'll do my best. On the afternoon of the 28 of Sept. we handled about 350 patients. The roads going to the front are all blocked and the patients who come to our hospital have been in the ambulance for over 24 hours. I saw one case where the blood soaked through the litter and dried and the patient was stuck to it. Twenty four hours without food or drink or blankets to keep them warm. Well on the night of the 28th we were ordered to move from Sivry La Perche to Cuisy. We arrived about 4:30 AM. I went to work right away. The Germans made a counter attack during the night and had driven the boys back about 5 kilometers, and the Americans were making a stand in the town. And stand they did. There are not many shells falling near us then. I was within 200 yards of the line. Gee, but I was scared. Bullets sure have an awful sound. Even tho I knew that the Germans were close, it did not bother me much because the old 39th Infantry was between them and me.

We put the hospital up on the side of the road and went to work. We walked right out into our backyard and picked them up and carried them in. We were closer than the first aid station. We put out a big red cross and about 10 AM on the 29th a Jerry came over the lines and photographed us. They never shelled us. We were busy all the 29th [of September] but the Infantry kept going ahead. During the night the French moved a battery of four 6 inch guns alongside of us. They kept us awake all night.

On the 30th Jerry took their picture [of the guns] and on the night of the 30th I was sitting in my office when the gas shells begin to drop all around the hospital. As I reached for my mask my eyes began to burn. Unconsciously I began to blink and stopped going for my mask. Then I got it with my lungs. God but how that did burn. Then I got my mask on. My armpits began to burn and then between my legs. My eyes [were] still burning like fire and my lungs hurt so much that I could scarcely breathe. Daniel[1] sent me to bed. That boy sure did look after me. "Gas" paste [was] put all over me but still it hurt. On the 1st of October I had a fever. On the 2nd it was 103.8.° I saw it myself. On these two days the Germans bombarded the road with high explosive. A Major, a lieutenant and 17 soldiers were killed by a shell which struck the 306 F.H. just across the street and

---

1. Private Guy R. Daniel

Chapter 4. Gassed

then on the evening of Oct. 2nd about 7:30 PM, I got mine again. A shell hit outside of the ward tent. It dug a hole, tore down the end of the tent and moved me from my litter clear across the tent and piled me on top of a couple of men.[2]

I was knocked unconscious. When I came to, I was in the Evacuation Ward. Sgt. Fisher was looking after me. He told me what had happened.

I was very nervous and was sent to E.H. #6 at Souilly. The men who slept in the same tent with me at the Recruit Camp, Camp Greenleaf were in this E.H. #6. I sent for them and they came in to see me. Then to [the] French Gas Hosp. At 5 PM Oct. 3rd I was carried out and put on an American Hospital train. They are sure swell cars. I will tell about as much of it as I can remember. The bunks were arranged lengthwise in three tiers. The car is loaded in the center. There are 48 bunks to a car. The orderly has an office in the little room at the end of the car. I slept all night. We rode all

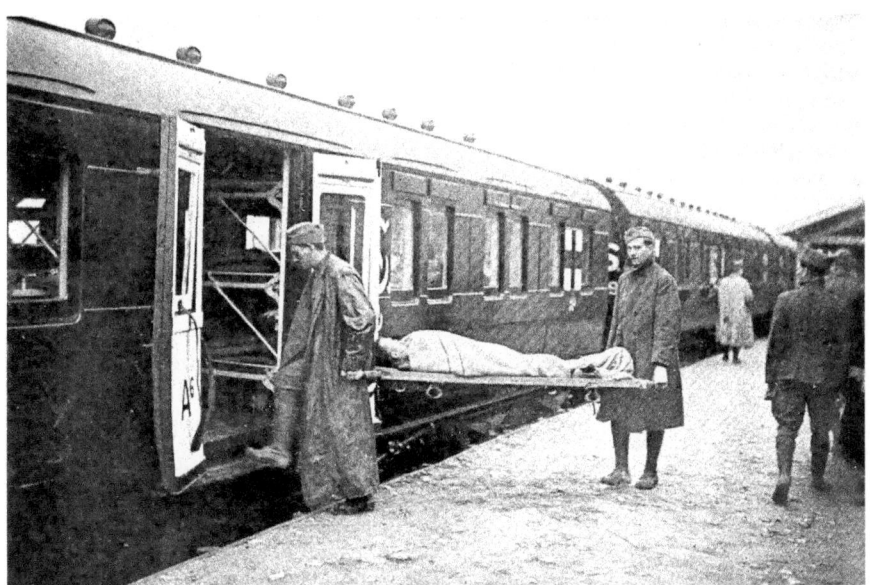

Loading the wounded aboard a hospital train (*The Medical Department of the U.S. Army in the World War*, Vol. VIII, fig. 9).

---

2. From the symptoms that Sergeant Brown describes, it appears that the agent that he was gassed with was mustard gas. "Gas Paste" (which was known as SAG paste—"gas" spelled backwards—was the treatment for mustard gas. It was a Vaseline-like paste that would be rubbed on the affected area to soothe the wounds and prevent spreading. It did not promote healing or prevent infection. The best treatment was to keep the area clean. (Source: http://roadstothegreatwar-ww1.blogspot.com/2015/02/fighting-mustard-gas-with-sag-paste.html)

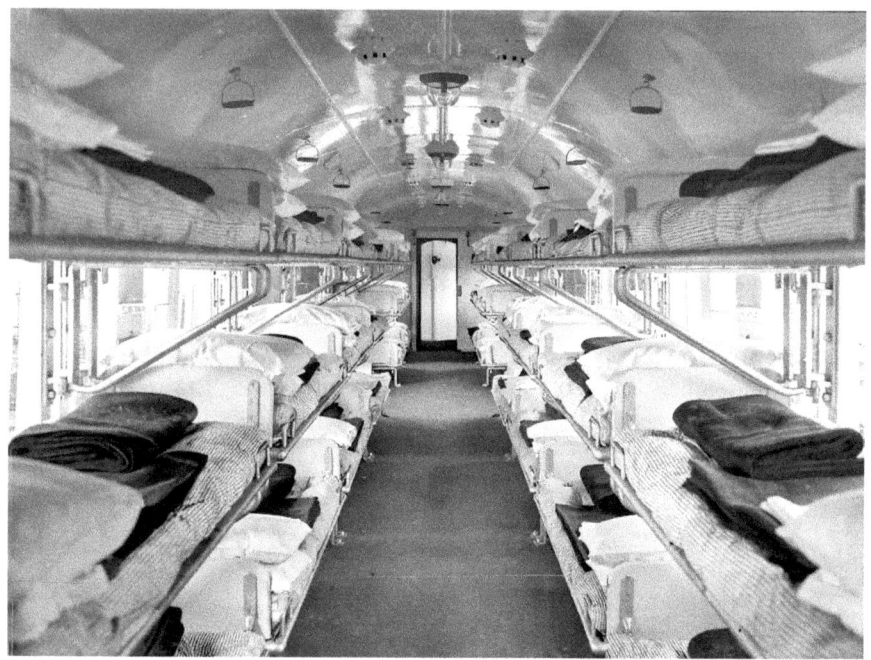

The interior of a hospital train, https://www.steampicturelibrary.com/p/121/no16-ambulance-train-ward-carriage-april-1915-15148800.jpg.

the next day and night and arrived at the B.H. [Base Hospital] at 2:30 AM on the 5th. I was put into a ward for gas patients. I was there about 12 hours when I was moved to the pneumonia ward. I don't remember much of the next two days. I was out of my mind. Then I began to feel better. Awful weak tho. Finally I got an appetite and then I got clothes and I was allowed to walk around the ward. I wrote home. I did not tell them about how sick I had been. My eyes still bothered me. I was weak and very nervous. I shook like a leaf. I kept getting better & better. I got a job helping the nurse and then Lieut. George Curran gave me a place with him and I was put on Detached Service with B.H. 50.[3] I suppose that means that I have seen enough of active service for this winter.

Well we get three good square meals every day. A good clean bed and when we go to bed we do not have to worry about being bombed or grabbing our gas masks. Oh how good it feels to rest again.

Today there was not much work. I received a letter from Evelyn Auspack. It seems strange but when I arrived at Camp Greene, I received my

---

3. Captain George L. Curran was from North Adams, Massachusetts. See the appendix for his profile.

first letter there from her. In France the first letter was hers and now that I hit the B.H. again the first letter was from her. Gee but no one knows how much mail is appreciated.

11 November 1918

Mesves, France

News came tonight that all fighting has actually ceased. It sure is a hard thing to believe. I have a copy of the New York Herald telling of it. The German prisoners are just as happy as we are. I imagine that my division is going into Germany. I do wish I was able to do that with them for I would like to see some of that country.

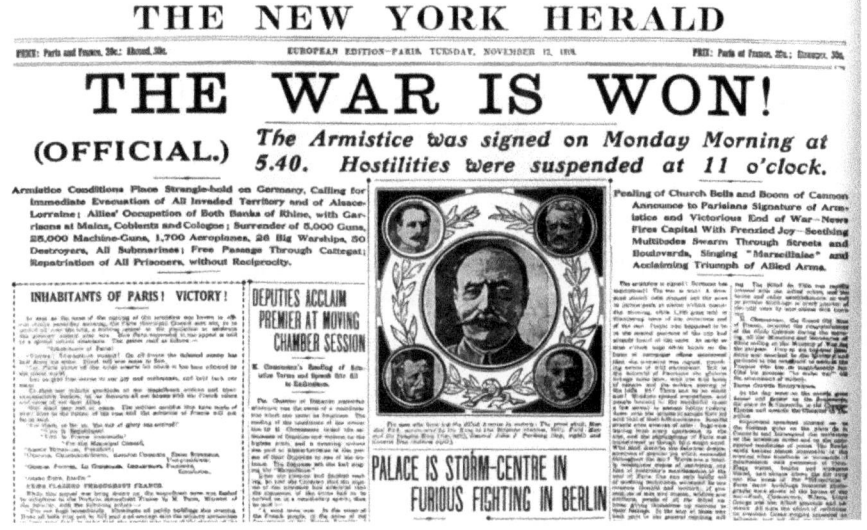

The New York Herald, November 12, 1918. This is probably the issue he is referring to in his diary entry of November 11.

Letter from Sgt. Brown's father

5 A.M. French Time 10 A.M.

Monday Morning Nov. 11

At 3:45 this morning I awoke and heard a whistle in the distance, then another and then I called mother and Alan. Alan dressed in fact—we as well as everyone in the neighborhood got up. Alan is off to town I suppose to see the celebration. I don't imagine there will be much work in Phila. to-day. I went down to Darby about 4:30 and some men came parading from Collingdale with a band. I don't know how they ever found a band here at this hour of the morning. This of course is a celebration of the aged, the infirm, the young and last but not least of the slackers and draft dodgers. Of course the real celebration will come when the boys come back from the Battlefield with the wound stripes and the European service stripes on their arms. Hope you are well enough by this time to be where you can see the real celebration at the front.

Dad

[Written faintly in pencil]

I never saw so many bonfires as I see this morning on my way in town. Even now at 6:30 am I have not seen a paper and no one has told me a word but I knew as I did when I heard the first whistle that it is all over and that the Dutch signed up as he was ordered by his Master-Marshal Foch.[4]

26 November 1918

Mesves, France

Received a letter from Maj. Phillips who said that Field Hospital #33 had been moved up into Germany. Gee but I sure wish that I were up with them. Old Walters wrote to me too. He has been made sergeant. I am glad of that [as] he sure does deserve it. Maj. Phillips said that he shipped my trunk on the 20th.

Am still working for Lieut. Curran. I write the history of the patient's disease. It is from these histories that the Ward Surgeon makes his diagnosis of the case.[5]

I am in an awful fix. I can't be sent to my division because it is gone to Germany. I can't get attached to this outfit because I am a noncom. I am a casual again and that sure is a Hell of a thing to be. It generally means, no place to sleep, no eats, no coin and no clothes. I sure am S.O.L.

I received 42 letters yesterday. They are from all over the world. Two were from Marian and several from home.

Now that the war is over, I suppose that I shall have to go back to writing about ordinary everyday affairs. There are lots of things which I went through and saw that I have not written down. When they happened they seemed quite commonplace but now and I look back, they seem quite novel.

---

4. Marshal Ferdinand Jean Marie Foch was a French general and marshal of France, Great Britain, and Poland; a military theorist; and the Supreme Allied Commander during the First World War.

5. Base Hospital No. 50 was a part of one of the largest and most important hospital centers. This hospital received both surgical and medical cases and was a special hospital for compound fractures and joint injuries. The total number of sick and wounded treated was 7,399, with 1,135 operations. The normal bed capacity of the hospital was 1,000; in a crisis it expanded to 1,950. "History, Base Hospital No. 50, A. E. F.," by the commanding officer of B.H. 50. From the Historical Division, S.G.O., Washington, D.C.

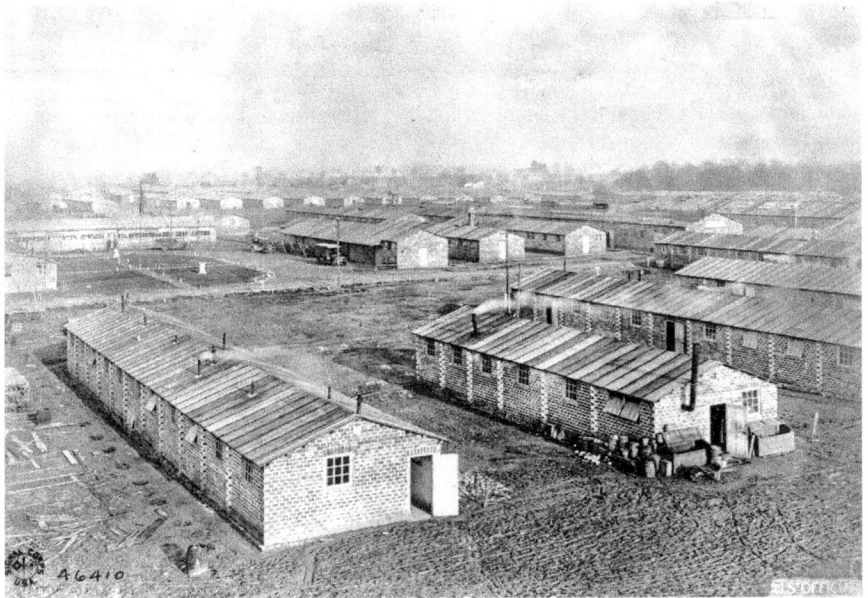

Base Hospital No. 50 at Mesves-Bulcy (U.S. Signal Corps #46410).

I received word from home that some school books of mine had been sent to me. I sure do wish they would come. I have lots of time on my hands.

Today I received a package of candy from Harrod's in London which mother and aunt Helen had sent to me for my birthday. It was one box of butterscotch, two boxes of licorice drops, one can of sardines. The candy sure is good.

I have not eaten any of the sardines yet. The box has a picture of Lord Kitchener on it. I showed to a German prisoner here and he told me that in Germany they say that Kerensky & Kitchener are the same man.[6]

November 28, 1918

Mesves, France
THANKSGIVING DAY

---

6. In 1914, at the start of World War I, Lord Kitchener became secretary of state for war for Britain. One of the few to foresee a long war, lasting for at least three years, Alexander Kerensky was a member of the Russian Provisional Government. His government was overthrown by the Lenin-led Bolsheviks in the October Revolution. He spent the rest of his life in exile in Paris and New York. (Source: Wikipedia)

The connection mentioned by the German prisoner was possibly propaganda voiced by the German government.

Well Diary we spend another Thanksgiving Day away from home. Next year we will sit down at our own table with the rest of the family (I hope).

But today we give thanks and I don't growl—and here is my prayer of thanks:—

Oh Lord, I thank thee hast given us peace from war; that thou hast read the prayers of the whole world. I thank thee for the protection thou gavest me during my trip across the Atlantic. For thy protection during that time I was at the front, and my recovery from my illness. My thanks for the health of my parents, my brother and the rest of my family.

I ask thy blessings upon us all. I asked that we shall soon be united again and that we may so live during the balance of our lives. In godliness, peace and prosperity.

And this I ask in Jesus' name—
Amen

We had a Thanksgiving Dinner, long to be remembered—Turkey—"beaucoup" of it. Cake, candy, nuts, filling, oh everything. I had all that I could eat.

I have had the blues for the past three or four days—Tonight I am going out for a walk. I may be able to lose them.

Letter to family, November 28, 1918

I think that I know you well enough to know that you were wondering what I am doing today. I got up this morning and ate a great big breakfast. I worked till 11 o'clock and then I waited for dinner. And such a dinner—Had turkey, as much as I wanted and I could have had more. Potatoes, filling, nuts candy. Then I slept all afternoon and tonight I went into town.

I went into a French café. Some dump. Low ceiling, one oil lamp, dirty and smoky. The tables crowded with American soldiers and French girls. The girls were all smoking and the air was so thick with smoke that you could scarcely see the other end of the room. You could hear English, French, Spanish and Italian and a mixture of all four. At the table next to mine and there were two French girls one American soldier and a French civilian. A drunken person came in and started arguing with them. Then the fight began. Bottles, glasses and everything else went flying across the place. I sure did enjoy the fight after being here without any excitement for so long a time. Then the military police came in and put a stop to the fun.

It rained as usual tonight and I walked about four miles in the rain so I am pretty wet.

Monday, December 2, 1918

Mesves, France

Thanksgiving night I went to town to a French Café to share a bottle of

Chapter 4. Gassed

wine with a buddy. The place was a dirty, evil looking place when I opened the door I could not see the other end of the room for cigarette smoke. One smoking oil lamp lighted the whole place. The place was crowded with American soldiers and French women. Soon I secured a seat. My table was next to one occupied by two French girls, an American soldier and a French civilian. I soon found out from the talk that the women were all prostitutes, which did not surprise me at all because the prostitute among the women of France is the rule not the exception. A drunken Black soldier tried to pick up the French girl and offered her two francs. She threw his money back at him and hit him with a wine glass. The Black soldier called her a dirty bitch and started after her. A great big white southerner hit the Black soldier and said, "Well she may be a whore but she is a white woman and you treat her as such." Then a regular race war was started. I got out quick—

Nothing new lately [I] am still on the job.

December 5, 1918

Mesves, France

We had an inspection this morning by Chief Surgeon, A.E.F. Everything went O.K.

I received a Bill of Lading for the trunk. It was shipped from Cuisy (Meuse) to Pouilly (Nievre). I am going to go over tomorrow and see if the box has arrived.

We had a little excitement here. Three days ago our chief nurse was taken ill. During the night she presented the hospital with the daughter—quite an accident—usual lies and explanations are being offered all around.

The way which the American nurse has acted in France is a disgrace to the Army and the American people (not all the nurses). They run around with the married officers to little private hotels [and] stay out all night with them and be about half dead the next day.

I had a letter from Ireland today. We are still having the usual six days rain out of seven. The mud is awful.

Today, Lollipop, who used to be with me in F.H. #33 came over and brought me two cigars and a pair of russet kicks [knickers]. It is the first pair that I have seen for six months.[7]

December 7, 1918

Mesves, France

I walked to Pouilly yesterday afternoon. I found my trunk. Got it, put it

---

7. Lollipop may be Private Stephen Poplawski, who was transferred from Field Hospital No. 33 to Ambulance Company 28 of the 7th Divison. (Source: Ohio Soldiers in World War I)

on a train, came to Mesves. Lugged it about a mile to camp. Opened it. Everything I own except my helmet, my revolver and my old 69 cent fountain pen is in there.—Gee Walters Old Man, a thousand thanks for packing it.

I went to a lecture on bacteriology last night given by Lt. Szymanski [Szypkowski] who was a member of the American commission to Serbia to study typhus fever.

Letter to family, December 7, 1918

I have not been paid since the first of September. My funds consist of about 3½ francs and two one dollar American bills. By the way, one of them is of the new Federal Reserve issue. I have never seen one of them before.

It is winter with you but I suppose with us is more like the fall. The only kick I have is that it rains almost every day. Have not read any papers since about Sept. 20th. I am anxious to know what the American papers said about the end of the war. Did you celebrate much? We are all looking to home now and the sooner the better.

Sunday, December 8, 1918

Mesves, France

I had a swell time going through my footlocker yesterday. It was like old times again. Finished my work yesterday morning. Yesterday afternoon I gave a patient 14 oz of normal saline solution by hypodermic injection. The fellow was pretty well gone-he died last night at 6:30. There is one thing I noticed and that was how tough the skin was. I found it comparatively hard to push the needles into the flesh. After I got through the skin, I found out it was easy to push the needle.

It has been three months since I have received any pay. Just at present my finances include two one dollar American Bills and 3½ francs French money. I have another cold in the head and a bad cough—I am going to stop smoking and see if that helps—I slept fine last night. Got up and finished my work early this morning. This afternoon I am going out for a walk and enjoy the country. The sun is trying to come out and if it does-well there are mighty few places which rival a clear French Day.

Later

Feel better now. Took a swell walk and learned something about the history of this part of the country. It was right here that Joan of Arc fought the English.

There was a big bunch who left here for the states today.

9 December 1918

Monday Mesves, France

When I went to work this morning the Lieut. told me that after I had

Chapter 4. Gassed

finished yesterday, Lt. Col. Jolson came in to see a patient. He asked the patient if Lieut. has seen him. The patient said no. Then the Col. went to the fellow's record and found that it had been written up. Then there was war for sure. I worked all day as usual. I worked pretty hard too. Tonight I am going to go to another lecture.

Tuesday, December 10, 1918

Mesves, France

I went to the lecture last night but the officer who was to lecture did not come. It is to be held tonight instead. I was talking to Miss Lighthall today. I told her that I had seen some Frenchmen kissing each other. She said, "Oh Sgt. please show me how to do it." The joke is on her.[8]

I saw something today which was a surprise to me. It is quite a problem to get rid of the coffee grounds here. The Yanks looked things over and now we are building a road with them. I went to a lecture by Maj. Fick tonight.

Friday, December 13, 1918

Mesves, France

Sent in my application for a transfer to this organization yesterday. For the past three days I have been making out pay books for the patients in the wards.

The wardmaster in ward 5 was sent to a hospital in Nice. Lt. Fick was going to give me that job but Major Fick of Seattle, Wash. needs someone to assist him and Lieut. Curran has promised me that place. On Wednesday night I went to a lecture given by Capt. Plummer.

I am reminded of the little incident which occurred last August at Fere-en Tardenois. We had a gas alarm and one of the boys could not find his gas mask. He was pretty badly scared. He began to cry and go around and shake hands with all of us and bid us Good-bye. We sure did feel sorry for him because he was a dead one for sure, but it was a false alarm, and we sure did kid him about it.

Letter to family, December 15, 1918

I am attending lectures here at the hospital. They are given by some pretty big men. Three subjects are being given just at present. "The Heart" The man who lectures is

---

8. Alma Evelyn Lighthall, RN, 1889–1966. More information about her can be found at https://basehospital50.blogspot.com/2018/01/alma-lighthall-macadam-rn-anc-1889-1966.html.

named Fick. He is the man who looks after all heart diseases for the Mayo Bros. His lectures are great. He surely can talk. "The Ear Nose and Throat" is another given by Capt. Plummer. He has studied all over Europe and in American universities. Then we have a lecture by physicians whose name I do not know. He was sent to Serbia by U.S. government to find an end to the Typhus Epidemic. So you can see by that they are pretty big men and they know their dope.

My lieutenant has promised me a trip to Nice. I am looking forward to a few very good times while I am over here. I suppose you know Nice is on the Riviera. Is quite near Monte Carlo and therefore on the Mediterranean close to Italy. Gee! I am for that. Of course it is like everything else tho, you never can tell.

Today has been the first clear day we have had for weeks. Perhaps it is because the President is here. The French people sure do think a lot of him.

Wait until I get home. I have a bunch of stories to tell you. Of course you can expect to have a bunch of lies just as the Civil War veterans used to tell. After I tell you the stories I'll tell you whether they are the truth or not. Reminds me of a true story that happened at a Epaux, France, just about 6 miles north of Chateau Thierry. We had a gas alarm. Was in the middle of the night and we all put our gas masks on. There was one fellow would could not find his. He surely was scared. He came around with tears in his eyes and shook hands with us and bid us goodbye. But it was a false alarm and he still lives to be kidded about it.

The customs of this country are funny to an American. A couple of weeks ago I had my trunk shipped from Verdun to this hospital. It came alright but when I went to the R.R. station, they sent me to the mayor of the town. I gave him a paper about the size of a newspaper and he gave me one about the same size. Then I took this to the American police who signed it. And then I had to go back to the R.R. station and get my box. I came to this town from the town where I live on the train. You don't have to pay any fare on the train. All you have to do is get on. You never see a conductor.

Monday December 16, 1918

Mesves

Took a walk yesterday as I had the afternoon off. Did not sleep very well last night. Everything going along Jake. [?]

I want to write a couple of poems

My Father

    Could I forsake these rugged ways
    These paths where now I walk with men,
    And lie me back to childhood days,
    To be, in body born again—
    From out this heart I call my own,
    From out this soul, forever free
    You are the father, you alone,
    I should ask God to give to me.

    When you're far away from home and you're feeling kind of blue,
    When the world is topsy-turvy, nothing sets just right for you.

Chapter 4. Gassed

Yuh can sneer at all your troubles, an yer cares yuh never mind
When you've really had a letter, from the Girl yuh left behind.[9]

"Hommes 40, Chevaux 8"

Roll, roll, roll, over the rails of France,
See the world and its map unfurled, five centimes in your pants,
What a noble trip, jolt and jog and jar
Forty we, with Equipment C, in one flat wheel box-car
II
We were packed by hand, Shoved aboard in teens
Pour little oil on us, And we would be sardines,
III
Rations? Oo-la-la and how we love the man
Who learned how to intern our chow in a cold and clammy can
Beans and Beef and Beans, beef and beans and beef
Willie raw, he will win the war, take in your belt a reef.
IV
Mess kits flown the coop, cups going up the spout
Use your thumbs for issue forks, And pass the bull about.
V
Hit the floor for bunk, six hommes to one homme's place
It's no fair to the bottom layer to kick 'em in the face.
Move the corporal's feet out of my left ear
Lay off, sarge, you're much too large, I am not a bed sack, dear.
VI
Lift my head up please, from this bag of bread
Put it on someone else's chest. Then I'll sleep like the dead.
VII
Roll, roll, roll, yammer and snore and fight
Travelling zoo, the whole day through and bedlam all the night.
Four days in the cage, going from hither hence
Ain't it great to ride by freight at good old unc's expense.

Wednesday, December 18, 1918

Mesves, France

Yesterday was another of the rare clear beautiful days for which France is known. Worked hard all day and last night. I went for a walk to Mesves. I was sick with diarrhea all night. Did not get much sleep. It rained all day today. Worked all morning and in spite of the rain, I went for a walk. Went to Bulcy and saw a ruined castle. Came back in time for supper.

Went to a lecture tonight by Capt. Copeland Plummer on the nose and ear. Now I am home ready to go to bed. Miss Shiedy went to Nevere

---

9. The poem "Getting Letters" continues for several pages and was taken—as was "Hommes 40, Chevaux 8"—from *Stars and Stripes*, an Army newspaper published for the troops.

[Nevers] and brought me some lace. Cost $14 and it is handmade and sure is pretty. I don't know what to bring home for Dad and Alan.

Letter to his father, December 18, 1918

Yesterday was clear and beautiful as only a clear day in France can be. But today—rain again. It did not affect me as is generally does. I took a long walk through the rain and mud and visited an old castle. I don't know its name neither do I know its history but I sure did enjoy seeing its courtyard and its towers and the house itself.

Before I came to Europe I had an idea that these castles were great big immense affairs. But just the contrary is true. The one today for instance it occupies no more space than does the little church on Hillside Avenue [Collingdale] and it is only as high as a two story house.

I have been shopping too. One of the nurses went out with me to the house of an old French woman who makes lace by hand. I am going to bring some home to mother. Well yesterday she had almost finished the set of three pieces. It is to be worn on the woman's night gown. I can't spell name but I think it was camisole. That is one piece. The other two pieces are for the sleeves. It has taken this woman nearly eleven months to make these three pieces and they cost me $14. I hope you don't think I am wasting my money but it is real handmade lace. And you know how much mother likes anything like that. The nurse who nursed me when I was so sick is taking care of the lace for me. She is surely a Princess and I want to take care not to forget her.

Thursday, December 19, 1918

Mesves, France

I sure am tired. Worked hard all day. Captain Plummer sent for me and I have been going through the wards and having the men sign the payroll. Burt was over to see me today but I did not get a chance to see him.[10]

Saturday 7 AM, December 21, 1918

Well diary, I worked all day yesterday with the payroll, having it signed. As I pass through the diphtheria ward I saw "Ike" Lindley. He has "Dip"—Poor kid-he sure was sick. After I ate supper I came to my tent and began to take it easy. Suddenly I remembered that it was lecture night. I went over to the eye clinic. We sat there until about 7:30 when Capt. Plummer came in and told us to go to the morgue for a lecture. I have been dreading going there ever since these lectures started. When we got to the morgue there was a Black man on the slab. He was opened

---

10. Perhaps he is referring to James Burt from his Camp Greene days.

up and all the organs of the trunk were shown and explained to us. I got weighed too while I was there; 147 pounds. Evidently I have not lost any weight.

Letter to family, December 21, 1918

They are evacuating this hospital fast and I don't suppose it would be long until we are all home and there will be not be an American soldier left in France.

Today I was over in the kitchen and in the butcher shop. I suppose you know the soldiers are always kicking about their food. It makes no difference whether it is good or bad. Well I never saw so much food piled together all at once. We feed 2200 here at the hospital. Big piles of beef. It takes six men at night and three in the day to cut the meat. Four men during the night and four man all day to cut the bread. The place where the tin cans are dumped would make a city dump hide its head in shame. They have built a road half a mile long in the middle of August with the coffee grounds.

We are getting ready for Christmas. We have been out gathering mistletoe. It grows in great abundance here. I never saw so much. I miss the holidays and the cold weather. Oh for a nice cold snappy day with the Mercury about 20°. This summer in December doesn't suit me at all.

Tomorrow is Sunday and we have mashed potatoes and roast chicken for dinner. I suppose that you know we live from one week to the next looking for the chicken. Did I ever tell you about the wooden shoes that I have? Got them near Chateau Thierry last July and have been lugging them all over the country. I wish I could trust them to the mail.

I went to another lecture last night. It was held in the Morgue. I saw a body opened. Something which I have never seen before. It was quite instructive and interesting. That is as interesting as such a thing could be. I hope I don't have to go to many more such lectures. My idea of the many organs of the body has been greatly revised.

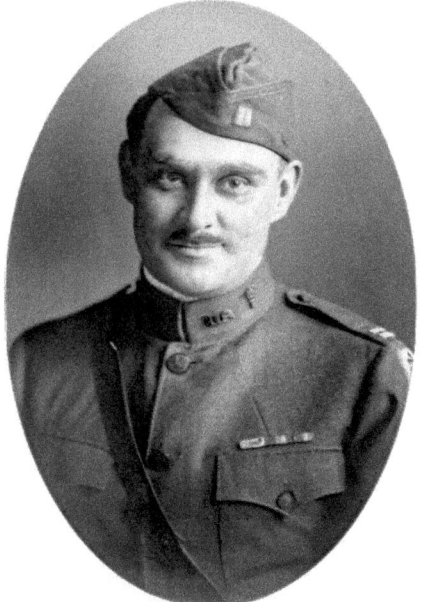

Lieutenant Curran, General Medicine, Base Hospital No. 50 (courtesy of Jane Curran-Meuli).

Sunday, December 22, 1918

Mesves, France

Pretty busy all yesterday, signing the payroll. Went to a movie show last night. Today another big bunch of men went to Nice for a vacation. Lt. Curran said that he needed me too much just at present to send me. I have been pretty busy all day making out their papers.

Sunday night and all is well. Took a long walk this afternoon along a country road. It reminded me of the march that we took when my company was relieved from duty in the Chateau Thierry sector. We were relieved two days before we left. On the night of August 12, I think it was, we left Chateau de la Foret and marched all night to St. Eugene which is a little S.W. of Chateau Thierry—we got lost. We marched about 22 miles from 9 PM to 7:30 AM. The last 5 miles was hell. It was all uphill and at a pace much faster than we have been using.

Then I had to stay up and look for the straglers [sic] and it was past noon before I went to sleep. I just laid on the ground and I was asleep in no time. I had to get up at 6 o'clock to make out some reports. No grub was being cooked so I went about a mile down the hill and paid five francs for two eggs and a piece of bread. Got to bed about 10:30. Next morning we got up at 3 AM and continued to march to Montmirail. Gosh it was hot. And I stumbled along the road. My gun belt cut into my hips. My canteen was dry. My lips parched and I spit dirt at every step. I could not march in the road. My place was on the side of the columns and how I remember when I passed those depressions which are used to drain the road, how I cursed them.

During my walk today I passed over some depressions and they made me think of my march last August.

I walked through an immense vineyard today. They do not allow the vines to grow more than two feet above the ground. They are supported by bean poles. These are planted in rows just like just corn and in the fall all leaves are removed from the plant and the vines are pruned.

Last letter I had from home was almost a month ago and was dated a month before that so I have had no word from home since last October. Gee, I would like to hear from them.

Tuesday, Dec. 24, 1918

Christmas Eve

We are having a celebration tonight and a patient wrote this for me. I sure do appreciate it. The Chinese means that he and I and another chinaman are comrades.

I wish I could describe the way we celebrated this Christmas Eve. It was a mighty poor specimen of what we do if we were home. But I do not think the most gifted man would have enjoyed himself much more than we did. We put a Christmas tree in the ward. One of the men dressed himself as Santa Claus and gave us all a stocking. The stocking contained a pound of candy, a pound of nuts, two packages of cigarettes, a box of matches, a

Chapter 4. Gassed

package of chewing gum, a handkerchief and the other sock. It sure was Christmas Eve.

Here is a buddy of mine's address.
Wm Bert Skinner[11]
Berwyn, Nebr.

Letter to Father, November 25, 1918

Merry Christmas Dad

I wonder if I can picture you reading this letter? You and mother and Alan.

Alan is jumping around. It seems as if he does not know where to go or what to do. He is thinking of the date that he has tonight and that he does not want anyone to know about it for fear they might make fun of him. You make so much noise that Rex raises up his head to see what the trouble is. Finally he says in a rough voice, "What's in that letter" and you just smile and go on reading.

Mother is sitting in a rocking chair and thinking (now I am going to be selfish)— she's thinking of me and wondering why I can't come home soon and what I am doing. Well I'll tell you what I am doing on Christmas morning. I am thinking of this letter at home. Then I look on the other side of the room and there is Dad. He is the chap to whom I am writing this letter. He turns aside from his newspaper and reads this letter. I can even see you smile and hear you chuckle. You wonder what I am doing with my little 3x4x9. Well I'll tell you I am stuffing it in me just as fast as I can. I am sitting in my office right next to a fine fire keeping warm and smiling across to the chief nurse who occupies the room with me. I am at peace with everybody and I am happy and content and glad to be alive.

How is the candy and nuts and fruit that you are eating? Chicken or turkey this year? You are not going to enjoy it half as much as I am going to enjoy mine because I am hungry. I am at every meal for that matter. Well now that the Kaiser has quit and that the circus is over we can forget our troubles and the scrap and we can look old and call ourselves the European War veterans and think about the time that we will have when we sit around the country store or stand on the street corner squirting tobacco juice on the ground and lie like hell about the regiment of Germans we captured just exactly as our grandfathers did for us when we were little fellows.

Well Dad once again "Merry Christmas" and may the new year see my return to good old U.S.A. Let me put my feet under Mrs. Brown's table and I'll never ask for anything else. Tell mother I said Merry Christmas to her and do the same to the kid.

Love to all—Leland

---

11. William Burdette "Bert" Skinner was a member of Company G of the 355th Infantry and was part of Base Hospital No. 216. He was possibly a patient at Base Hospital No. 50, where Sergeant Brown was a working patient. In the records of the Army Transport Service, Private Skinner returned to the United States aboard the USS *Rijdam* in April of 1919. Then he was attached to Convalescent Company 144 as a walking patient, apparently recovering from influenza.

Letter to Family, December 25, 1918,

My thoughts have been with you all up today. It seemed like Christmas to me even though I see mud and rain in place of snow. We decorated the ward yesterday with mistletoe and put up the Christmas tree. We trimmed it with paper and cotton and I made some of those little trimmings like we used to make for our tree when Julian was living. One of the boys dressed up as Santa Claus and the Red Cross gave each of us a sock. We had a pound of candy, a pound of nuts, two packages of cigarettes and a box of matches, a handkerchief and the other sock. One of the nurses gave me a handkerchief. Then we were all issued a pint of red wine and we sure did enjoy ourselves. Today we received two more boxes of candy—chocolate and gum drops. We had "beaucoup" turkey and it makes me homesick. I wondering how you spent your Christmas. The last letter from you was dated on my birthday [October 20] so you see I have had no fresh news from you for over two months.

I am getting worried. I hope that you have escaped the "flu." It is only lately that I have understood how very serious it was in the states. So many have died that I almost hate to get any news from you. I surely have prayed that you keep well. Coming home seems farther off than ever. They don't seem to be in such a terrible hurry to get us back. We are not very busy at the hospital. The wards have very few patients. There's just not much to do and time hangs heavy on our hands. It would be a saving to the government and a pile of pleasure to me if they would discharge me and send me home. I haven't even received the Philadelphia papers since those dated September 18–22. There must be a car load of mail waiting someplace for me. To sum up the whole letter in a few words I'll say, "I am homesick."

26 December 1918

Christmas was great all day. Of course I felt blue and we had mud and rain instead of snow and sleet but that is the chances we all take. I should worry!

I am going to be an optimist instead of a pessimist. Dad wrote me today and here is his saying

All right Daddy, if you can smile so can I grit my teeth and smile too. We had plenty of turkey yesterday and I received 16 letters. I think that I can groan and stand it a little while longer.

Letter to family, December 26, 1918

Today I received five letters from you [and] the last one was mailed Nov. 15th. I have not received any pay since Sept 1st but don't send me any money. It costs you money and I can't get any cash and I pay something too. I think I am a good enough soldier to scrape along broke if I have to. I am going to write each of you an installment in the letter. First part is an answer to mother's letter-next-Alan's-then Dad's.

I am sorry that you did not receive much mail from me during September and the first of Oct. I know I wrote you quite often because there were lots of new places and

Chapter 4. Gassed

things that I saw during that time. However as long as we hear from each other once in a while and there is some short interval between, it will give us something to talk about when I get home again. I would sure like to be home right now.

I was thinking about that little room which you used to call mine, and I was planning how I was going to fix it up. Of course I have not seen much of it and I do not remember just where the windows are. Yet I always look to it as mine. I hope you're taking care of all things that I have sent home since I came into the army. Each and every one of them mean a whole lot to me. Above all please take care of my camp pictures.[12] *They're all I have to remember my trip to the south with. It does not look as though I will come home very soon. I am afraid it will take longer to take us back then it did to bring us across. We have no British ships now and the English handled about three quarters of our men when we came to Europe. I have received about one batch of papers since I came to this hospital. I have not received my Christmas box yet and do not expect to before the middle of January. I have been sort of dreading to get mail from you because almost everyone has had news from home that someone near to them had died with the "flu." I am afraid that some of you might get it.*

I sure glad that the "go to H___" outfits do not impress you. To me they are a bunch of "Johns." I have seen too many of the world's best soldiers to be impressed with them. They are the men you see parading on Chestnut St. during peace times with big red ties and loud socks. That is a gang that once you belong to you are never able to get away from. Of course you will hear lots of blowing when these men get back to the states but the real men, the real fellows who did the fighting and who were up the front will have mighty little to tell you about themselves. They will be bored to death when you talk to them about it. The truth is just before I left the line there was mighty little to interest me. Extraordinary things to you were ordinary and everyday occurrences to me. I tried to tell you of such things as would interest you. When I wrote in my diary the things that would make interesting reading to other people were not what I wrote down. There was mighty little enthusiasm with the men on the line. They just looked at a fight as an ordinary day's work. They worried more about their "chow," their pay and the place where they slept than they did of the Boche bullets. I heard one man saying that the only real night's sleep that he had since coming to France was a night before he went over-the-top near Verdun. He told me you didn't give D___ what happened, he was going to sleep. I know that there were times when we would get bombed and I just woke up and turned over to go to sleep again and expressed my thought in language plain and clear that the blooming Dutch had disturbed my sleep.

When I came back here in the S.O.S.,[13] *I met a very different bunch of men. Those men had never seen a firing line, never seen them get hit and die, never heard a shell shriek or bomb burst. Had never seen a hand grenade or worn a gas mask in a gas attack. They are the ones are making heroes of themselves and are getting away with it too because the people in the states did not stop to think that France is a fairly big place and that some men never get closer than 2 or 3 hundred miles from the front.*

I am anxious to hear _____ talk about the war. I have bet that he has been over-the-top a dozen times. I never have but I have been close to it. He is located at _____ and that is about 100 miles from the coast and he will stay there until he is sent home.

---

12. Photos he took while he was at Camp Greene, North Carolina.
13. "S.O.S." refers to service of supply (see the glossary).

I have sewed my 6 mos. service chevron on my coat sleeve. Sewed on the same coat I wore when I was home last May. I still have that coat and will not part with it if I can help it. I have a little bar which I wear too. It was given to me at the French hospital where I was sent to from my own outfit. It is given to every wounded or gassed soldier who passes thru a French hospital. It has a star on it and is quite a fancy little addition to wear. And there is another thing, I have met quite a number men who have won the "Croix de Guerre" and the much prized D.S.M. medal but none wear the medal. They all wear the less conspicuous ribbon.

I had a letter from Eddie Shinn today. I think he is sorry that he did not get a chance to come over and see the fun. But he didn't much at that. [?]

France is a heck of a country when it rains and the "greatest show on earth" soon gets to be monstrous, Especially when the roads are shelled so heavily that it was impossible to bring up food and we had to live on corned Willie. Gosh I hate that stuff. It sure will go hard with the fellow who invented it if the soldiers ever get a hold of him. I would also say that it is surprising how much nourishment you can get out of a piece of hardtack and some corned Willy. We lived on it for about two weeks once. That will be some experience to tell you about when I get home. And when I tell you about how we got it, you will laugh. Well Daddy aren't you glad that I enlisted and came over. And you too mother, aren't you? And you would have been ashamed if I had stayed at home.

December 29, 1918

Mesves, France
Sunday

Received some copies of the Philadelphia Bulletin of September 30, October 1 and October 2 yesterday and a copy of October 22 came today. I sure do enjoy reading them. They tickle me about the letters they publish from soldiers over here. It must be an honor for you to get drafted in the states. I see where some lucky duke was the holder of the first ticket to get drafted. If he had any pep he would have been in it long ago. Then I see where Sgt. Bell of Mobile Unit No. 2 has grabbed all the credit [and] the citation from Gen. Pershing. Because he stayed on duty while under shell fire. How about the other poor devils who belonged to the unit and who are not so well-known. Nothing new with me. Same old story—rain and mud and then more rain.

Letter to family, December 29, 1918,
A.P.O. 798

Have received quite a number of [news] papers during the past three days. I sure do enjoy reading the bull about the army and the soldiers. That tickles me. I see where the son of the Ex District Attorney Bell of Phila. grabs all the credit for working his hospital under fire. More power to him if you can get away with it.

It must be an honor to be drafted by the way the papers read. I see where some guy in

Chapter 4. Gassed

Philly gets one of the lucky numbers and he has picture in the Bulletin. If the war was still going on I should say, keep it up. It looks fine.[14]

I understand that this base hospital may go back to the states about the middle of February. I hope that they do and that I shall go back with them. I will unless I am attached to some unit which will stay over here longer than that.

10:15 PM December 31, 1918

Mesves Bulcy, France

Well diary we are at the end of another year. This time far away from home. Tonight brings up memories of past years. I remember when I was a little fella I used to go to bed early and then my father would call me just before 12 o'clock and I remember how the whistle and bells would frighten me but I would soon become so sleep[y] I would go right to sleep. Then as I got older I stayed up to see the old pass into the new. I remember one New Year's eve that I had an electric bell connected with a battery and I celebrated that way. Then last year, I shall remember that well. I left Charlotte N.C. on December 30. The train was delayed by snow and cold and it was noon on the 31st when I got to Washington. I had stood all the way up. Then Sgt. Eddie Huid and I took the 1 p.m. train for Philadelphia. It reached Darby at about 7 PM. I remember we laid out on the railroad there for about an hour but I couldn't get off. About 9 PM on December 31, I got off at West Philadelphia. First I ran to a telephone booth and called Woodland 633W.

"Hello that you Marian?"

"Yes"

"Do you know who this is?"

"No-oh yes hello Joe."

"This is not Joe."

"Oh no, hello Herb."

"This is not Herb."

"Yes it is you Herb, you can't fool me I know your voice too well. You call me up too many times."

---

14. Sergeant Brown is talking about Sergeant First Class De Benneville (Bert) Bell, the son of the former Philadelphia district attorney, John C. Bell. Bert Bell was the captain of the University of Pennsylvania's football team when he enlisted and was attached to Base Hospital No. 20. Both Bell and his commanding officer, Lieutenant Colonel John B. Carnett, were cited for bravery, as were two nurses and a private. Perhaps Leland felt slighted that his hospital work was not so honored. In 1933, Bell was the cofounding owner of the National Football League (NFL) team the Philadelphia Eagles. He was creator of the NFL amateur player draft and acted as the league's commissioner from 1946 until his death in 1959. In 1963 he was posthumously inducted into the Pro Football Hall of Fame.

"I tell you this is not Herb (sarcastically)—I just came in from North Carolina!"

"WHAT LEE?"

"Nobody else"

Then the Fire-Works

That sure was great trip and I saw Eddie Thorne then too. And in front of me I have a letter from the Azores dated in September 1918 and one from him from Philadelphia dated October 1918.

This year has seen the death of my grandmother. She has been gone for 7 months now.

Yesterday I became so disgusted with this place tonight that I asked to be shipped out. Today I was called before the Disability Board. I was placed in A class. There is the barest chance that I will be shipped to my division. I may never see my outfit again, but all that I ask is that I am placed in the Fourth Division again. F.H. 33 is now at Saalsberg [Saarburg], Germany. I sure do hope in a couple of weeks I shall read this in Germany and smile.

Letter to family, December 31, 1918

Looks like I am about to see some more of France. This hospital is evacuating all of its patients. I went before the examining board again today and I was placed in class A1. That means that I am physically a perfect soldier again and all ready for another campaign. (I wonder if it will be with the regular Army in Russia?). I may leave here any day now so if there is any time between this letter and the next, it will be because I am traveling and I am not able to write. I am hoping to be sent back to the Fourth Division, but it's only a hope. I do want to see Germany. I hope that my next letter will be written while on my way to Germany and that the next one will tell you that I am there. I would have cabled you a "Merry Christmas" but was afraid it would scare you to death. Did Washington ever notify you that I was in the hospital? I have noticed that lots of casualties which I reported were never published.

1919

2 January 1919

Mesves Bulcy, France

I went to bed at about 11:30 and just got to sleep on the night of

Chapter 4. Gassed

December 31, 1918, when four or five men who sleep in the tent came in about half drunk and proceeded with the aid of several bottles of cognac to finish the job. Gee, I never saw such a wild happy bunch. Finally a fight started and the whole bunch joined in. Then at midnight they made up again and came over and tried to get me to drink some. Well it ended up by one fellow pouring some on my head and saying, "If you won't put it on the inside you'll put it on the out." And they got a hold of some revolvers and proceeded to shoot around the tent. I finally went to sleep. The party continued.

Yesterday was a sort of a holiday. Seven A class men were shipped out but I am still at Mesves Hospital Center. I received my first letter from Dad direct from home to B.H. 50. Then I walked to La Charite and bought some flowers for Lieut. Curran and walked home with them. After that I was so tired that I went right to bed.

Today has been more or less quiet. I had a letter forwarded to me from Aunt Helen where she told me how she celebrated Armistice Day, Nov. 11th, 1918.[15] [obliterated text]

Letter to his father, January 2, 1919

I read yours of November 11th [to]day. You sure must have enjoyed yourselves. There must have been a bunch of rejoicing in the states. You got up early in the morning and I had almost finished my work for the day. When I was back in the states I used to think as I went to bed, "Well it is just about time for the boys in France to be going over-the-top." Thank God that is all over now.

It surely was awful while I was at the front but I'll tell you now that it is all over and I have come thru. I will say that I would not have missed it for anything. A fellow never knows what fear is until he dodged the big ones and has heard the little ones whine. I am not looking forward to my journey away from here with any great amount of pleasure for it means three or four days travel in a box car with hardtack and corned Willy washed down with water that [tastes] like chlorine of lime. However, if I am a class A1 soldier, I can pull thru with it as I have done dozens of times before.

5 January 1919 Sunday

Mesves

I went to La Charite yesterday for Lieut. Curran. He has quite a case on Miss Russell, one of the nurses here. I bought some flowers for the Lieutenant and brought them back to the hospital.[16] Today there has been

---

15. Aunt Helen is Helen Nelson Brown, Leland's father's spinster sister (1878–1948).
16. Lieutenant Curran and Claire Russell eventually married. For additional information about Colonel Curran and Miss Russell see the appendix.

absolutely nothing doing. Just hanging around the place. Had mail from home. Mr. Holland (Leland's preceptor in pharmacy school), also wrote to me. Mother said that Eddie Thorne had been out to see her.

Letter to family, January 7, 1918

I am having all kinds of hope of leaving here this week. All the men who have left here so far have been shipped back to their old organizations except a few casuals who never belonged to any definite organization. I find much to read that interests me in the papers you sent. There is a boy here from the 28th Division and he finds much more war new[s] to interest him than I find to interest me.

I think that in one of my letters I wrote and told you about all the towns I had been in up to the 1st of Sept. Well we left Liffol-La-Petite then and came by way of St. Dizier to Bar-le-Duc. It was an all day and all night journey on motor trucks. About 3 A.M. we reached a little town 5 km from Bar-le-Duc called Varincourt [Vavincourt]. At first we had our hospital in some aeroplane sheds and then we moved a little closer to Verdun in a woods.

That sure was an awful place. It rained the whole time we were there and when we left we had to build about ¾ of a mile of road to get the trucks through the mud. Then we moved to Haudainville [which is] N.E. of Verdun. We stayed there only one day when we moved back along the Meuse to a little town not far from the line at San Mihiel. I have forgotten its name. Then that drive started. We were really shut off from news of any kind and this battle was different from any other Battle in that no patients came back. We only handled one patient in that scrape. He claimed to be gassed but he was simply nuts.

I did take my reports every day up to Haudainville and pass thru the city of Verdun to do it. One night my motorcycle was stolen but the reports had to be in so I set out on foot. I walked to the main road from Bar-le-Duc to Verdun and asked the Military Police, or rather told him that I had dispatches for Haudainville but had lost my motorcycle. He said he would furnish me transportation. The first machine to come along contained two French officers but that made no difference to that MP. So in I went and I was taken up to Verdun. I had to walk from there to Haudainville.[17]

Well we left that place and went to Lemmes [which was] S.W. of Verdun. Then overland in [a] truck to Sivry-la-Perche and there to Coincy [Cuisy] from where I was sent back to Souilly and then down to this place.

I had a letter from my company this week. My division (4th) is holding the Bridgehead at Coblenz and my company is about 12 kilometers from there at a place called Kaisersechen [Kaisersesch]. So I may be able yet to see the Rhine.

Wednesday, January 8, 1919

Mesves Bulcy, France

Still here at base 50. Monday a bunch of men left here who belonged

---

17. The distance from Verdun to Haudainville is about 3.5 miles.

Chapter 4. Gassed

to the 1st Division. Today a bunch left who belonged to the 2nd Division. I hope that my Division soon sends for its men. I sure do want to get away from here. These men so far have all gone to their companies. Today Lieut. Curran gave me a separate room to sleep in. It sure is nice in there. We have a stove and everything else for our convenience in there. Hope I go to Germany soon—

Thursday, 9 January 1919

Mesves Bulcy, France

I like my new room very much. Had a good night's sleep last night. Got up this morning and did a little work. There is not very much to do tho—They are sure sending out the cases now. The wards have very few cases in them now. It hardly seems possible that the war has been over for two months. Had a letter from Mrs. Maxwell today. Men from the 36-37-91 Divisions were sent away from the hospital.

Saturday, 11 January 1919

Mesves Bulcy, France

I went to La Charite this afternoon but before I left I reported to the A class tents. I was told that I am ordered to report to Toul. After I came back from La Charite I drew two blank[et]s, extra shoes and socks—winter underwear and soap and towel. Then I came back to my quarters and found a package Aunt Helen sent to me from London through John Wanamaker. It contained two boxes of candy and 1 pound of almonds.

Went out collecting souvenirs and found the cartoon which is shown on the next page.

Compliments of Miss Ethel E. Roche A.N.C. without her permission.[18]

Letter to family, January 11, 1919

I am going to leave this hospital tomorrow and go back to my Division. From there I go to Toul. It is quite a big town up near old Lorraine. There I hope to be sent back to number 33. I suppose that I will ship via boxcar because that is the way we travel in this country.

[End of the letter books]

---

18. Ethel Emily Roche was a nurse from San Francisco who was attached to Base Hospital No. 50. "A.N.C." refers to the Army Nurse Corps.

Thursday, January 16, 1919

Toul, France

I left the Mesves Hospital Center on Sunday, January 12. I had my things packed in a barrack bag. It sure was full and mighty heavy too. Pvt. Davis helped me with it. Down at the station I was put in charge of a boxcar and Burt from Field Hospital #33 was in it. Sure was glad to see him. We left Mesves Bulcy and went to Nevers where we stayed until about 1:30 AM. Next day we passed through Is-Sur Tille and about 5 am we reached Toul on Tuesday morning. We were given a pack and full equipment.

Yesterday I had charge of the detail which cleaned the Y.M.C.A. in the morning and in the afternoon I policed another Y.M.C.A. Got two packages of cigarettes and some cakes from them. Today I had a detail which policed up a building. After that I went out on the drill field and drilled the rest of the morning. This morning breakfast was rotten. The rest of the meals we have had are sure good.

I met some men from Pennsylvania National Guard who had been prisoners in Germany. They are fat enough now but they tell me they sure did starve for a while.

Friday, January 17, 1919

Toul, France

I went out with a detail and policed up of some barracks. This took nearly all morning. This afternoon I went out in the drill field and drilled all afternoon. I am eating much better than I was. There is a large aviation field near here. The aviators are the best that I have ever seen in France. They fly the machines in all kinds of weather. Rain or shine, there are dozens of machines in the air. They loop the loop. Do those spins. One fellow swooped down—cleared our head by a foot and swept up again. We all fell flat and held our breath.

22 January 1919

Toul, France

Still at the replacement barracks. There's nothing happening now. It is simply a case of wait for orders. We don't even know whether we are to go to Germany or whether we are to be sent to some other division or to the states. I hope Germany. I would like to stay there for a while before I go back home.

Chapter 4. Gassed

Sunday, 26 January 1919

Toul, France

Got up early this morning [at] 5 A.M. Ate breakfast and put on a full pack. Marched to the station and sat there for an hour. Then they found that there was no room for us and marched us back to camp. Gee, but I was mad. We are going to try again tomorrow.

Chapter 5

GERMANY

Thursday, 30 January 1919

Kaisersesch

On my trip north I passed the night on the train without any sleep at all. I passed through Metz, City of Luxembourg and then on up through Germany proper to Treves. At 7:30 A.M. I arrived at Cochem. Loaded in a truck and went on to Kaisersesch where I joined the outfit. Boy it sure is some place right on the top of the Eiffel Mountains. The boys gave me a royal welcome. Then I was sent into a private house to live. I like my place very much. Sgt. 1st Cl. Fisher is going to live with me. I have my old job back again. And I like it very much. I hit Germany on the 28th of January 2 A.M. in the morning.

Friday, 31 January 1919

Kaisersesch

Worked on the monthly reports all day today. Feel pretty tired tonight. This family consists of a father who is Burgomaster, his wife, three daughters 23–18–12 and two sons: 19–14. The eldest boy was in the German Army. Night before last the oldest daughter made me a 4th Div. insignia.

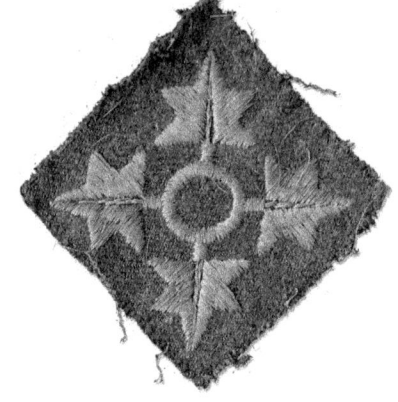

The 4th Infantry Division's shoulder insignia shows four ivy leaves for fidelity and tenacity. The ivy design is a play on "IV," the Roman numeral for the number 4. This was Sergeant Brown's shoulder patch. It was thought to have been designed by Major General George Cameron, the 4th Division's commanding general when the division was formed at Camp Greene, North Carolina, on December 10, 1917 (Carolyn Taylor Brown).

Last night she sewed it on for me and also put my chevron on and made my coat a little bit small in the back. She refused to take any payment for the work she did. There must be something in the wind.

Tonight when I came home from work, I went into my bedroom and found that my O.D. [olive drab] blanket had disappeared. Well I have not had a chance to look through the room as yet. If the blanket has disappeared I wonder where it has gone and why. In other words I am awaiting developments. I wrote to Burwell and Marian today.

Saturday, 1 February 1919

Kaisersesch, Germany

I.
I picked two dark roses in the beautiful time of May,
I picked them for my darling
O, what a joy!
I carried them to the window
where my darling lives
and waits for this gift
which he repays with a kiss.
Darling come, come,
Leave your house!
Darling come along,
out into the open.

II.
A youth with curly hair
Must go off to the military.
His farewell to his darling
Pains him.
His heart beats powerfully,
It gives him no peace
And as he leave he calls
Again to his darling.
Darling come, come,
Leave your house!
Darling come along,
out into the open.

III.
In the evening, the sun sets-11
On the far horizon.
The moon comes
To the birds in the forest.
I heard a bird singing,
It sang the whole night

From the evening until the morning
Until the day awakes.
Darling come, come,
Leave your house!
Darling come along,
out into the open.
—Käthe Ollig[1]

One of the girls in the house where I live wrote this is my diary. She is looking over my shoulder now and trying to read this. She said she understood it but she don't. Now she's trying to translate it into English by using a great big vocabulary.

Maj. Phillips went to Coblenz today. I finished the monthly reports.

Old Fisher pulled a gag that he was sick and when I came to the house he was holding hands with one _____. He sure is a heartbreaker. He has more girls than any other man in the company. You don't believe me ask Alice. She lives at Acy, France. She wrote him. "Why you go away and make me no explain. Why is it."

[End of Diary]

---

1. This folksong is widely known in Germany, especially in the Rhineland where Kaisersesch is. It was originally written in German and signed by Käthe Ollig, presumably the person who wrote it in Sergeant Brown's diary and one of the young ladies living in the house with Sergeants Fisher and Brown. Translated from the German by Frank Hoeber.

Afterword

After Sergeant Brown's last diary entry, we know very little of his time in Europe. That final entry was on February 1, 1919, from Kaisersesch, Germany. His company did not sail to the United States until July 21, nearly seven months later. Since he was at Mesves, France, when his division moved into Germany, he was saved the rigors of marching to Kaisersesch (where his company was billeted). As he was a casual, he returned to his outfit in Germany by train and truck from France. We do have a fairly complete record of what the 4th Division was doing during this time. The following account of that period draws on Christian A. Bach and Henry Noble Hall's 1920 book *The Fourth Division: Its Services and Achievements in the World War* and the American Battle Monuments Commission's 1938 publication *American Armies and Battlefields in Europe.*

The division began its march into Germany on November 20, 1918. The Americans were to occupy the center section of the occupied territory, with the British taking over the northern section as it was near their base of supply. It was natural for the French to take command of the southern area of Germany, which had been part of France from 1792 to 1815; French sympathies were thought to still exist there a hundred years later.

General M.L. Hersey, who was in command of the 4th Division, had the following general orders read before the troops before the division began their occupation of Germany:

> In the great offensive movements which have ended the present conflict, the men of this division have taken a conspicuous part. Your valor has been demonstrated. You have helped to change the map of Europe. You have made history. The American Army to-day is confronted with a greater task than that of defeating a martial foe. We are now to occupy enemy territory; we are to help build a new Government to take the place of the one we have destroyed; we must feed those whom we have overcome; and we must do all this with infinite tact and patience, and a keen appreciation of the smart that still lies in the open wound of their pride. If we, while animated by just pride of achievement, eliminate from our demeanor the overbearing of the conqueror; if we

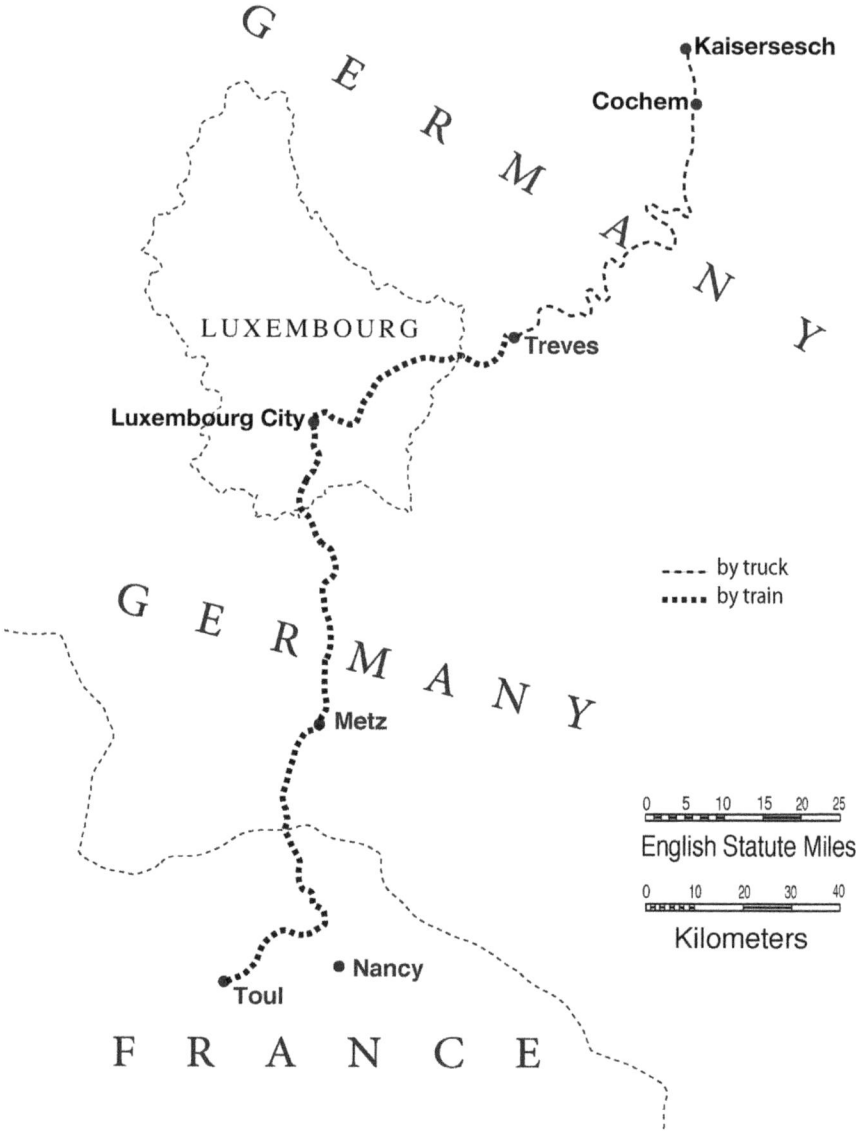

After leaving Base Hospital No. 50 at Mesves-Bulcy on January 12, 1919, Sergeant Brown traveled by train to Toul, France, arriving at 5 a.m. on January 14 and passing through Nevers and Is-sur-Tille. He remained in the replacement barracks at Toul until January 27, when he traveled by train to Cochem, Germany, passing through Metz, Luxembourg City, and Trèves. He then continued by truck to Kaisersesch, Germany, where his company was serving in occupied Germany. He arrived there on January 19, 1919 (map by author).

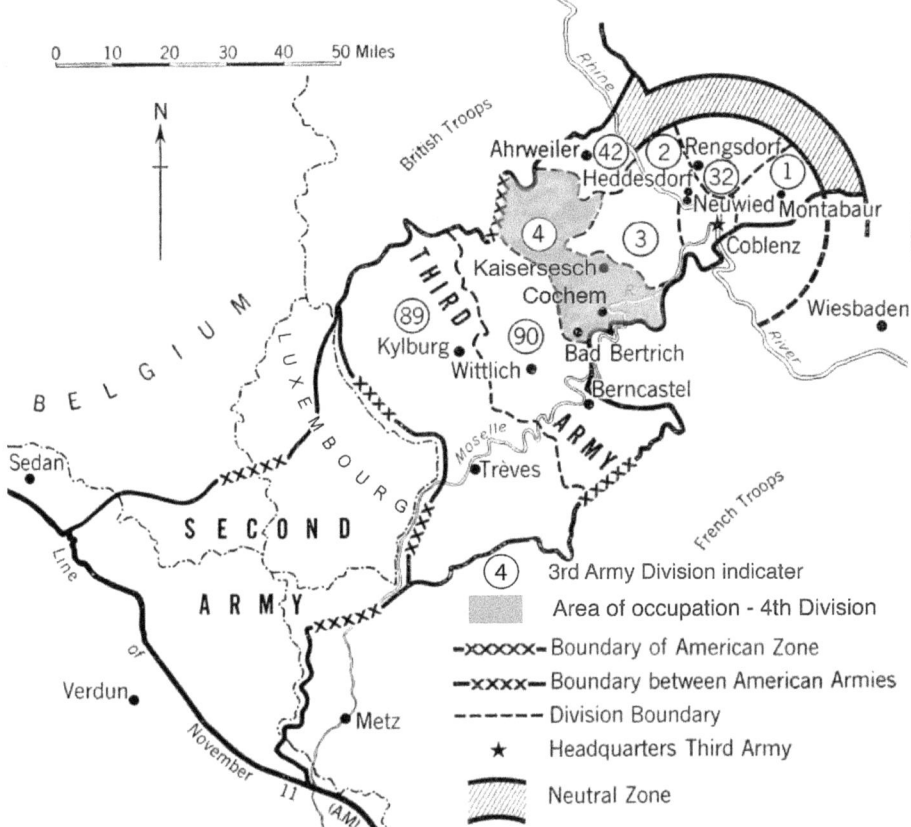

Map of the American area of occupation in Germany on December 21, 1918, with additions (American Battle Monuments Commission, *American Armies and Battlefields in Europe: A History, Guide and Reference* [Government Printing Office, 1938], p. 489.

make them see that our perceptions include not only an appreciation of our sufferings but of theirs as well; if we convince them that our sole aim in entering the war was to make implanting in each German breast a deep and abiding respect for America and American institutions. The war is over. No useful purpose can be served by continuing, after war has ceased, the hatred that war engenders. As we have helped to destroy the old Germany, let us help now to build up a new Germany. The work on which you are about to enter is an exceedingly difficult one. The humiliation and sting of defeat caused a proud people to feel a natural bitterness toward its conquerors. The feeling is intensified when the conquerors enter its territory. Women, children, old men, will show their resentment toward the troops of occupation. You must meet all manifestations of this bitterness in a dignified and soldierly manner. Show by discipline, self-control, generosity and helpfulness that the American soldier is as chivalrous as he is invincible. The people of the United States are watching you to see how you will measure up to the requirements of this task. Meet the test as you have met all other tests.

On their way north through country that had once been French, they moved through Conflans, where the citizens welcomed the Americans by showing the French tricolors. These had been hidden during the German occupation. In addition to the French flag, there were many handmade American flags with from 10 to 20 stripes and from four to 40 stars that the soldiers enjoyed as evidence of the citizens' efforts and appreciation.

Then they passed into Lorraine, which had been returned to France. Lorraine had been taken from France in 1821 by the Germans. Decorated arches had been erected by the inhabitants for the soldiers to march through, bands played, and local girls danced. In the area of Hayange and Serémange-Erzange, they rested from November 23 to December 1. They celebrated Thanksgiving Day on November 28. There was no turkey, but they were well fed just the same. They slept in real beds and enjoyed the pleasures of a liberating army. But within a day or two, they were to cross over into Germany, where they would find themselves in the country of the enemy and where their conduct had to be proper. They were told that they should not fraternize. Many realized that it would be a great adventure that could hold many risks. Some thought they would be killed by the Germans or segregated from them. On December 3 the leading units crossed the Moselle and were on German soil, arriving without any fanfare or ostentation. Their welcome in Germany had been that of silent, staring faces. The field kitchens were particularly of interest to the children. In Lorraine the children had discovered chewing gum that the soldiers carried, but in Germany their tastes had turned to chocolate.

Before they got very far into Germany, a battalion of men was sent ahead to Koblenz to maintain order and perform police duty with the blessing of the local German authorities. The women of Koblenz were especially open in their hostility, and some men sneered at the men patrolling the streets. Things became more cordial once the soldiers frequented the shops, hotels, and restaurants.

Since the German people esteemed military officers as superior beings, casual relationships between the officers and the German people would cause a lessening of prestige. It was determined that the American officers were in Germany not to be friends with the Germans but as their military governors. They were told by their superiors that they had to be courteous but not familiar, refrain from giving or receiving hospitality or gifts, and cease any friendly relationships with the populace.

The route on which they were traveling was arduous. The weather was bad (sleet and rain) and the terrain rocky, with endless deep valleys and ridges to climb. On December 17, the march was accomplished. This march—of approximately 330 kilometers (205 miles),—was the longest march made by any American troops in Europe during the war.

The area that the 4th Division occupied was on the south of the Moselle River. It contained the districts of Cochem and Adenau, an area about 34 miles in length from north to south and varying from about 20 miles to six miles in width. It was a large and difficult area to govern as there were problems with communication and supply due to the steep hills and valleys.

The main headquarters for the division was at Cochem. The 77th Artillery and Field Hospital No. 33 were at Kaisersesch. Soon after the division arrived, arrangements were made for entertainment for the men, including sports such as boxing and football. Also at this time the 13th Field Artillery became motorized. The noise and smoke of the tractors hauling their loads over the hills amused and astonished the local populace.

When the Germans left the area that the Americans were to occupy, they instructed the various *Landräte* (district administrators) to cultivate friendships with the American soldiers. Their small friendly acts did not go unnoticed by the Americans. There was little overcharging by the shopkeepers. This was in contrast to what they experienced in France, where some thought that the Americans should pay for the war. As time passed, however, intimate associations with American soldiers led to friction, especially when girls or political differences were involved. This was not unexpected. The respect with which the Americans were initially treated when they arrived soon wore away.

Movies and variety shows arranged by the YMCA were available to the men. Boxing matches between the various divisions were popular. A so-called "flying squadron" of American girls was imported to convince the soldiers that "made in America" was the most desirable option. Whether they were persuaded is lost to history.

Along with these various entertainments, it was thought necessary for the troops to march and parade. It was difficult to find level ground for a parade area in this terrain. They were able to find a suitable place, but it took two days of marching in sleet and rain to arrive there. Still, they were able to parade for the army commander, General Pershing. Despite all of this, it was a reported to be a huge success and recorded in the division's history thus:

> Across the wind-swept field, on which patches of snow still drifted here and there, the long line of soldiers advanced, keeping perfect time with the band,

their steel helmets surging forward like a disciplined wave. The sturdy figures of the men, their smart marching stride, the wave after wave of olive-drab that rolled by, gave an impression of tremendous power that filled all with pride who beheld it. At the head of each regiment were the Stars and Stripes and the regimental colors, their folds sweeping back as the bearers marched forward. As they approached the reviewing stand, the bugles sounded; officers' hands went up to the salute; the regimental colors dipped; all eyes were turned to the General, and the moving mass passed on. Line followed line; the machine gun companies followed their regiments; the machine gun battalions followed their brigades; engineers, signal battalion, sanitary train. The condition of the ground did not permit the artillery to march past. The thoughts of many of those who viewed this impressive scene turned to the Marne and the Ourcq, the Vesle and St. Mihiel, and to the scenes of the great struggle in the Meuse-Argonne. The pride of achievement was written on the faces of officers and men alike. If many were missing, if many had paid the last full price of devotion to their country and their country's cause, their sacrifice had not been in vain. Here the 4th Division stood on German soil, a part of the victorious American Army, its task well done, its purpose accomplished. After the march past, the men were told to break ranks and group themselves as closely as possible about the reviewing stand. Speaking from the top of the stand, General Pershing addressed the officers and men of the Division. In clear, ringing tones he told the story of the entry of America into the war, at a time when the Allies needed help and of the services rendered by the 4th Division. He reminded the men that when they returned home they would be looked upon as leaders and consulted by their fellow-citizens on many matters of national importance, that the prestige they, as veterans, would enjoy in their respective localities would give them additional privileges and responsibilities and urged them to prepare themselves to play as worthy a part in peace as they had played in war. Then he told them what a fine thing it was that amid all the temptations offered to them overseas they could go back to their mothers and sisters, their wives and sweethearts, happy in the knowledge that they were clean. He paid a special tribute to the women of America, so many of whom had worked for the army, and he spoke of their great influence with the men. Then General Pershing did a thing which showed how much he was pleased with what he had seen. In all the addresses he had made to the troops after reviewing the other divisions the Commander-in-Chief had only made a passing reference to the appearance of the men. But to the 4th Division General Pershing said that he could not tell them how deep an impression their fine appearance had made upon him, and turning to General Hersey he congratulated him on the splendid body of men he had under his command. Loud bursts of applause welled up from the tightly packed thousands of soldiers, but General Hersey stepped forward, and raising his hand for silence, said, "Men of the 4th Division, under the providence of an Almighty God there was given to the United States in her hour of need the Commander-in-Chief who has just addressed us. Take off your war helmets and with thanksgiving in your hearts give three cheers for General Pershing, our Great Commander.

Afterword 137

Every helmet came off when the word rang out. There was a pause amid the bare-headed throng, but when the last words had left their leader's lips, the men of the 4th Division cheered General Pershing as he had perhaps never been cheered before. And when the men had ceased, the echoes and re-echoes came back from over the German hills. No man could have stood there unmoved by so heartfelt a demonstration of admiration. No man could hear those roaring cheers without feeling his blood run faster. If the men of the Ivy Division had won General Pershing's admiration on the field of battle, the opportunity had come at last for him to receive their tribute. And they gave it to the full.

In early April the 4th Division moved north to the Rhine to replace the 42nd Division, which was returning to the United States. This area was considered to be the prime area of occupation as it contained many wonderful small towns and health resorts for summer tourists. The accommodations were superior to what they had experienced during their previous occupation.

A system of schools was established for the soldiers in which almost a quarter of a million men participated. At Beaune, a large university was established for advanced instruction. There must have been a similar situation at the University of Poitiers, where Sergeant Brown, Sergeant Arthur Fisher, and perhaps others from their company attended classes. The certificate that Brown received for his attendance at Poitiers noted that it was for "les Étudiants Americains." Brown studied agricultural chemistry there.

The division returned from their occupation area to their port of debarkation by using German railroad cars that were retrofitted by the Army Engineers with the necessary facilities for food preparation. It is unknown whether Brown and Fisher accompanied their division from Germany or met up with them at Brest.

On their trip to Brest, the 4th Division traveled through Cologne, Aix-la-Chapelle, Namur, Mons, Arras, Amiens, Rouen, Laval, Rennes, and Saint-Brieuc. At Brest the division was quartered at Camp Pontanezen. On July 18, 1919, decorations awarded by the French government were given. The men were subject to a final medical inspection and delousing and received fresh underclothes and new uniforms if needed.

Most of the men of Field Hospital No. 33, including Sergeant Brown, sailed on July 23, 1919, on the SS *Minnesotan* from Brest, France, and arrived at Hoboken, New Jersey, on August 3, 1919. They were mustered out of the Army at Camp Dix, New Jersey, three days later. Some members of that field hospital had remained in France as they were still recuperating from medical issues such as disease or the effects of being gassed or wounded in combat. Incidentally, the Army did not classify being gassed as being wounded, and those who were gassed were no doubt disappointed to not receive wound stripes to proudly sew on their uniforms.

Of the approximately 117 known soldiers who were attached to Field Hospital No. 33, only Private Fred P. Eberle died overseas (of pneumonia). His death date was reported to be either December 7 or December 17, 1918. There is a brief biography of him in the Appendix.

In the diary, Sergeant Brown often expresses a wish to travel and see more of France. There is a hint that he did. In his photo album there are photos of Biarritz on the Bay of Biscay, the Cathedral at Reims, and other places in France. Found loose in the diary were admission tickets to the Eiffel Tower and several of the châteaus along the Loire Valley, close to Poitiers.

It may not be a coincidence that the diary ends soon after the recorded letters stop. Things seem to have been warming up between the sergeants and the girls of the German family they were living with.

Surely there were other letters home before his return to the United States on August 3, six months after his last recorded letter, but they are probably lost. It would have been interesting to have the correspondence that he received while in the service and the letters he wrote to people outside his family. With all the carnage of that war being reported in the local newspapers (there were four men killed in combat from his small hometown of Collingdale alone) and with Leland writing to family from his close proximity to the front, his parents must have been extremely concerned about his safety. This would have been expressed in their letters to him. But we are fortunate to have as much as we do.

* * * * *

Leland often told outlandish stories, and when confronted about them he would seldom reveal if they were true or not. There were three stories that I remember him telling about his experiences during the war.

The first was about how he received his five belly buttons, which he displayed at the slightest provocation. This happened—as he told the story, he would point to his bare belly with its five dents—when he was fighting the Germans in hand-to-hand combat on the battlefield and was bayonetted in his abdomen. Before the German could pull the bayonet up into his chest area (for a sure kill), another American shot the German dead, and Leland survived. The resulting scars made it look as if he had five belly buttons.

In fact, the "belly buttons" were scars from a lifesaving operation he had in the 1930s for a perforated ulcer.

The second story, which might have some credence to it, hearkened back to his time in recruit camp at Fort Oglethorpe in Georgia, when all the new recruits were assembled. The sergeant asked everybody with an eighth-grade education to take a step forward. Most did. Then he asked all those who had a high school education to take a step. About half of them stepped forward. When anyone who had a college education was asked to come forward, he was the only one to do so. The person in charge said that he was now the acting sergeant. According to his Army record, he enlisted in early October of 1917 and he wasn't made sergeant until more than five months later.

Perhaps during his preliminary training there was some similar situation where he would have been given a temporary higher rank during that time only?

When men were first brought to Camp Greenleaf at Fort Oglethorpe, Georgia, they were placed in a "Detention Group." After they were seen personally and their qualifications were evaluated, they were assigned to a company as a private, a private first class, or a noncommissioned officer (a corporal or a sergeant). This would have been a temporary rank when in recruit camp only. If what he states was true, he was reduced to a buck private when he came from Fort Oglethorpe to Camp Greene (as were all of the enlisted men who held a temporary advanced rank at Camp Greenleaf). Leland wasn't promoted to private first class until two and a half months after arriving at Camp Greene.

The third story was how he was awarded the coveted *Croix de Guerre* medal, given by the French Expeditionary Forces for bravery in combat.

As he told it, he was driving from the front in an ambulance with another soldier who had been wounded in the back. The road on which they drove came under enemy shell fire. He and his buddy thought that the safest place to be would be under the ambulance, so there they went. While they were still under the ambulance, a vehicle with French officers stopped and demanded to see their identification. The French took down their information and left. They felt for sure they would be court-martialed, for what they were doing was a serious, cowardly offense.

Some time passed, and there was an occasion for a formal ceremony in front of their company. Their names were called, and they thought they would be punished for their bad deed. The French officer, with tears running down his cheeks, hugged them and kissed them on both of their cheeks while pinning the *Croix de Guerre* on their chests. Leland and his fellow soldier didn't understand it until they were later told that they were being honored for "repairing an ambulance while under enemy fire."

This story is a bit hard to swallow. If one were under fire from artillery, it would make sense to get that ambulance out of there as quickly as possible. In a letter home, he does mention a similar situation: "We had to pass a place in the road that was under shell fire. A shell would come over and burst and then we would scoot for the other end of the road. It certainly was an exciting minute."

His diary stopped just when he arrived in Germany as part of the AEF occupation force. It was noted in the history of the 4th Division that on July 18, 1919, when the division was at Brest preparing to return to the United States that a number of awards were given to members of the division. These medals would have come with certificates of award, and none have ever been found in Sergeant Brown's belongings.

He did bring home that medal, but he doesn't mention having been awarded one in the diary. He does, however, write that when he gets home he'll "think about the time that we will have when we sit around the country store or stand on the street corner squirting tobacco juice on the ground and lie like hell about the regiment of Germans we captured just exactly as our grandfathers did."

Various Medals in Sergeant Brown's Possession After the War

The World War I Victory Medal

This was the medal that Leland received sometime after 1921 when it was issued to World War I veterans.

It was designed by James Earle Fraser in 1919. Fraser was better known for "The End of the Trail," sculpture of an American Indian on horseback and the design of the Indian head or buffalo nickel.

Sergeant Brown's Victory Medal is decorated with various clasps denoting involvement in the following campaigns:

Aisne: May 27–June 5, 1918
Saint-Mihiel: September 12–16, 1918
Meuse Argonne: September 26–November 11, 1918
Defensive Sector: for general service overseas in a war zone (not for a specific battle)

According to his Army records he was eligible for the **Aisne-Marne** clasp (July 18–August 6, 1918) but not the Aisne clasp. His application for the medal was incorrectly stamped Aisne instead of Aisne-Marne and therefore his Victory Medal has that clasp.

The obverse of the bronze medal features a winged Victory holding a shield and sword.

On the reverse the top is inscribed "The Great War for Civilization." A staff is on top of a shield that says "U" on the left side of the staff and "S" on

Afterword

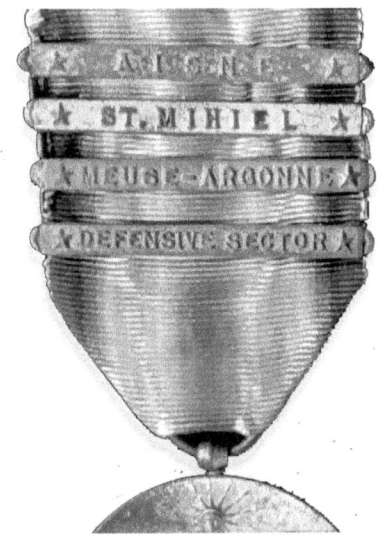

This is the medal that all World War I veterans received sometime after 1921. It was designed in 1919 by James Earle Fraser, who was more well known for the design of the Indian head buffalo nickel coin. Fraser also created "The End of the Trail," a sculpture of a Native American on horseback.

Sergeant Brown's Victory Medal is decorated with various clasps denoting involvement in the following campaigns: Aisne: May 27–June 5, 1918; Saint-Mihiel: September 12–16, 1918; Meuse-Argonne: September 26–November 11, 1918; Defense Sector: For general service overseas in a war zone, not a specific battle.

According to Army records he was eligible for the Aisne-Marne clasp (July 18 to August 6, 1918) but not the Aisne clasp. His application for the medal was incorrectly stamped Aisne instead of Aisne-Marne, hence his Victory Medal was so stamped.

its right side. Listed are the World War I Allied countries: France, Italy, Serbia, Japan, Montenegro, Russia, Greece, Great Britain, Belgium, Brazil, Portugal, Rumania [Romania], and China.

The Verdun Medal

This medal was created to commemorate the heroism of the defenders of Verdun. It is inscribed "ON NE PASSE PAS" ("They shall not pass"). Shown is the bust of Marianne, the national symbol of the French Republic. Originally awarded to those who served on the Verdun front between February 21, 1916, and November 2, 1916, the medal was awarded to those who served anywhere in the Argonne and Saint-Mihiel sectors between July 31, 1914, and November 11, 1918. The original and most commonly found version was by Vernier, but since supplies of this medal were inadequate, others created the medal and there are at least seven versions known. This was the medal that was in Sergeant Brown's possession.

The Croix de Guerre

Probably the best-known French decoration, this cross was awarded to all those who were mentioned in dispatches since the outbreak of war (August 2, 1914).

It was instituted on April 8, 1915, as an outward recognition for being mentioned in the order of the day of an army, corps, division, brigade, or battalion.

More than 2,055,000 were awarded. The reverse side bears the year 1914 together with the year in which they were struck (1915, 1916, 1917, or 1918).

"Sgt. Brown's medal" is dated 1914 and 1918.

If indeed he received this medal, he would have mentioned it in a letter to his family of December 26, 1918, in which he tells of others (but not himself) who had been awarded the *Croix de Guerre*. It would have also been accompanied by a certificate of award, but none was found in his papers.

There were other medals that were in his possession after the war, the *Médaille Militaire* and the *Légion d'Honneur*. Both were awarded by the French government, and it seems very unlikely that Sergeant Brown would have been awarded these medals as well as the *Croix de Guerre*.

* * * * *

Leland returned to the States in early August 1919, together with most of his company, aboard an Army transport ship, the SS *Minnesotan*. He was discharged at Fort Dix, New Jersey, on August 6, 1919. On his discharge papers it was noted that he was "gassed by the enemy on October 6, 1918." In his diary Sergeant Brown recorded that he was gassed on September 30.

He continued to work with Harry Holland, his mentor and preceptor, in Holland's drugstore. Holland, childless, took Leland on as his partner. Leland opened a second drugstore at 5561 Baltimore Avenue, also in West Philadelphia.

He maintained a relationship with his girlfriend, Marian, after he returned from France in 1919. This was evident through his album of photographs of them smiling together, but they didn't remain a couple for very long.

In September 1920 he married Asenath Rae Thompson Sutcliffe, a widow with a son, William T. (born 1916). He and Asenath had two more sons, Nelson H. (born 1922) and Herbert T. (born 1924).

In 1929 he and his wife adopted a daughter, Dorothy Marie, while his wife was having treatment for tuberculosis in California. The circumstance of her adoption was never made clear to his family. Asenath died in November 1931 after a long battle with tuberculosis.

It was also about this time that Leland lost his drugstores in bankruptcy due to the effects of the Great Depression.

Around 1930 he founded the Leland Brown Laboratories. At first it was a one-person operation in the rear of his pharmacy that analyzed blood and urine samples for doctors and hospitals.

At his offices at the Center Building in Upper Darby, Pennsylvania, he hired Elizabeth Brown (née Brown—no relation), 15 years his junior. She was a graduate of Pennsylvania State University and a former research assistant with Sharpe and Dome. Sharpe and Dome had ceased operation where she worked. Elizabeth decided to start a clinical laboratory but didn't have the necessary equipment. She asked Christopher Roos, her former boss at Sharpe and Dome, if they would part with the equipment that she needed. He said no, but also mentioned that he knew someone who would—and introduced her to Leland. She and Leland married in June 1933 and had two boys, Leland B. (born 1934) and William M. (born 1937).

In 1942, Elizabeth began studies at Hahnemann Medical College and received her MD in three years through the World War II accelerated program. She practiced throughout her life, specializing in the treatment of allergies.

During World War II, Leland volunteered in the U.S. Coast Guard Auxiliary. He was in charge of two picket boats at the beginning of his service and later commanded two Coast Guard tugs. The picket boats were used to patrol the Delaware River and Bay to thwart the German submarines that were wreaking havoc with Allied shipping along the Atlantic Coast. The family's private yacht was turned over to the Coast Guard without charge to be used for a similar duty. The tugs aided in ice breaking on the Delaware River. He received the rank of lieutenant, junior grade, in the Coast Guard Reserves. He also participated as a Civil Defense volunteer. For his service in World War II, he was awarded the World War II Victory Medal.

In about 1960 Leland expanded the laboratories into several branches employing as many as 10 employees. The company was sold in 1971. He was very active in the Rotary Club of Upper Darby, Pennsylvania, serving as its president in 1943.

In 1959 Leland and Elizabeth traveled to Poitiers, France, and met with the son of the professor who had been his teacher while he was in the service.

The family lived in Lansdowne, Pennsylvania, until moving in 1960 to nearby Wallingford, Pa.

He had emphysema for years, probably brought on by his having been gassed in France and being a chain-smoker.

Leland died in 1984 at age 90. Elizabeth kept her practice until soon before her death in 1994 at age 85.

Appendix A: Training to Be a Soldier in the Medical Department in World War I

The United States entered the war in early April of 1917 without enough trained personnel to fight a war. Lacking in most areas, they needed to greatly increase the medical capabilities of the Army. That required the training of medical professionals in battlefield medicine. Doctors were expected to tend to the soldiers' physical wounds, sicknesses, and psychological maladies. In addition to medical doctors, veterinarians and dentists were needed. So were ancillary personnel: men to drive and maintain the ambulances and trucks, feed and care for the mules and horses, prepare the food for soldiers and the patients as well as the many other sundry tasks necessary to maintain the various medical facilities in the war zone.

During that same month that war was declared, a Medical Officers Training Camp, called Camp Greenleaf, was planned at Fort Oglethorpe, Georgia. It was ordered that the students should not come until June 15, but the first 60 student officers arrived on the first of that month. On May 28 there were no completed buildings or tents on the site. By June 1, a building without walls was the only structure available. Soon, however, enough barracks, mess halls, and sanitary facilities were built to accommodate more than 650 student officers.

It appears that most, if not all, of the medical personnel of Field Hospital No. 33, both the officers and the enlisted men, were sent directly from their recruiting station to Camp Greenleaf.

It is assumed that all the enlistees were given normal Army basic training while at Camp Greenleaf. Enlisted men were attached to the Medical Officers Training Corps and were trained there to be soldiers and to do the necessary work required to run a field hospital. The medical officers and the regular enlistees of the Medical Department were trained both separately and together. As there were many different needs to be met in the medical organization of the Army, the personnel would be taught in different groups, both medical and nonmedical, depending upon their fields. The officers in training who were rated class A would act as instructors to the enlisted recruits.

Men who were experienced in pharmacy, nursing, or other medical fields were sent to the hospital group. In the beginning 100 medical officers from the Medical Reserve Corps and the National Guard served as instructors, but soon the most promising of the student officers were also doing some of the teaching. In this group were medical doctors, veterinarians, and dentists. There were men detailed for special instructions to learn other necessary related skills such as those of laboratory and radiology work. As to whether Private Brown, with his background in pharmacy, was singled out to be part of the hospital group directly is unknown.

There was also the motor group, responsible for the maintenance and driving of Army ambulances and medical supply vehicles. Those experienced as cooks or bakers, or those desiring to be cooks, would be so trained. This system was frequently not adhered to because it was often necessary to send whomever they could to fill all requisitions.

At Camp Greenleaf the most promising of the enlisted men were selected to become noncommissioned officers. As to whether Private

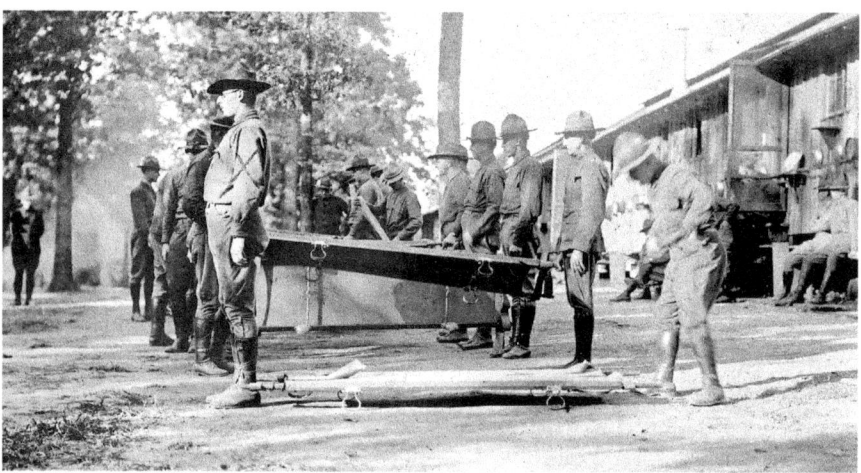

Litter drill at the Medical Officers Training Camp at Camp Greenleaf, Georgia, 1917. The soldier on the left of the photograph could possibly be Private Guy Daniel (courtesy of Lisa St. John).

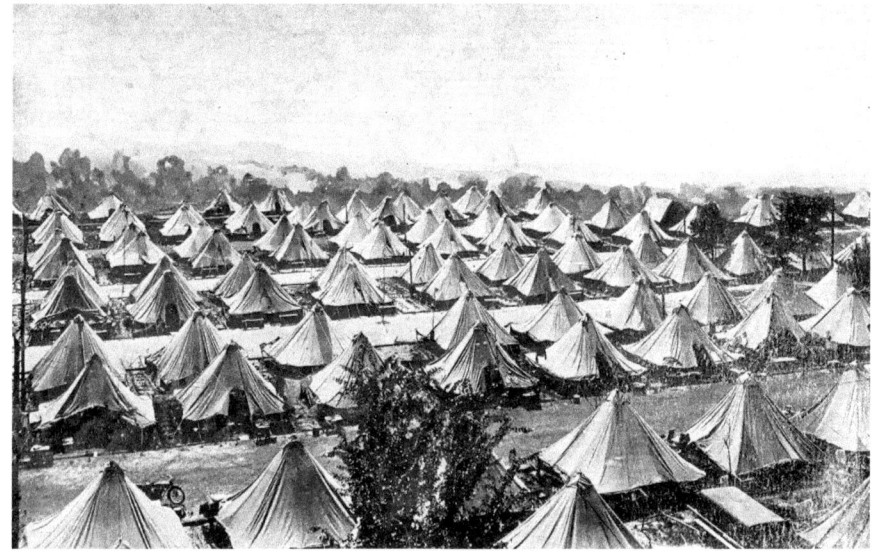

A postcard showing Camp Greene, North Carolina, 1917–1918.

Brown was in this group is unknown. Only medical doctors, veterinarians, and dentists would become officers with the rank of 1st lieutenant. The officers in training could be at Camp Greenleaf for up to three months. Private Brown was there in training for about two months.

On or about November 1, 1917, some field hospitals and ambulance companies were combined and then sent to camps for formation of divisional sanitary trains. This is when Private Brown's outfit, Field Hospital No. 33, went to Camp Greene, North Carolina. It was then attached to the newly formed 4th Division.

Camp Greene was named after Nathanael Greene, a Revolutionary War hero. It was a new camp constructed in 1917 after the United States declared war. It was built to train up to three Army divisions concurrently. In 90 days, 940 buildings were built on 2,300 acres near Charlotte, North Carolina. The camp was eventually expanded to 6,000 acres. At its peak, it was able to accommodate up to 40,000 men at one time. The camp was located in a southern area with the hope that weather there would be mild, but the winter of 1917–18 proved to be the worst winter in recent memory. The camp's tents were built on 16-by-16 foot wooden platforms and heated by stoves; there were eight men to a tent.

The land, consisting mostly of clay, was nearly impervious to water. When it rained or snowed, which was often, the ground turned to deep mud, causing conditions that made it difficult to move men and vehicles. It also became a health problem with the improper disposal of sewage. Soldiers often had to go without a shower or a proper toilet.

For almost six months, from November 1, 1917, to May 25, 1918, Field Hospital No. 33 remained at Camp Greene, where soldieers trained while waiting for the 4th Division to go overseas.

APPENDIX B:
THE PERSONNEL
OF FIELD HOSPITAL NO. 33

It appears that most, if not all, of the medical personnel of Field Hospital No. 33, including both the officers and the enlisted men, were sent directly to Camp Greenleaf at Fort Oglethorpe, Georgia. There they were trained in battlefield medicine. They were attached to the Medical Officers Training Corps even though only the medical doctors would become officers and obtain the rank of first lieutenant. The enlisted men were trained to be soldiers and perform the work required to run a field hospital. It is assumed that the enlistees underwent normal Army basic training while at Camp Greenleaf. Leland spent only a month there.

From Camp Greenleaf they came to Camp Greene, North Carolina, for the necessary advance training in the operation of a battlefield field hospital. This is where he began his diary.

In his diary and letters Sergeant Brown mentions more than 120 fellow soldiers in his outfit by name. Who were these men, and from what walks of life did they come? Were all the officers medical doctors? And were all the sergeants medical professionals before they enlisted?

Ancestry.com, Newspapers.com, school records, and various libraries were invaluable sources of information about the soldiers of Field Hospital No. 33. The archivists at colleges and universities that individuals had attended were helpful resources.

The official Army records of the personnel were lost in a fire at the National Personnel Records Center that occurred on July 12, 1973, in St. Louis, Missouri. The tragic loss of these records made the research difficult. The existing records of the U.S. Army Transportation Service, which transported the soldiers to and from Europe, survived and was very useful to the research. They contained the full names of the personnel of Field Hospital No. 33, their service numbers, and the addresses of each soldier's next of kin, which provided clues to pre-enlistment places of residence. From the passenger list in a few cases it was possible to determine which soldiers had deserted just before being shipped to Europe. Even though their names were obliterated on the passenger list, I was able, with a little luck and digging, to be able to find the names of the three deserters: Phillip Enwright, LeRoy Shearer, and Walter Wigington. Enwright and Wigington must have turned themselves in or been arrested, as they later rejoined Field Hospital No. 33 in France. No further information about Shearer was found.

Pennsylvania had an added information source. The World War I Pennsylvania Veteran Service and Compensations files are a series of records created in 1934 when the Commonwealth of Pennsylvania offered bonuses of up to $200 to World War I veterans. Ohio and Maryland and other states had less detailed records of their World War I veterans, but, nevertheless, these files were very helpful for they included each soldier's service number, where and when he enlisted, the military campaigns in which he participated, the various units he was attached to, and what ranks he attained and when. In a few cases, such as that of Lieutenant Dick, the Pennsylvania Compensation Files included letters written home and photographs. Unfortunately, not all the soldiers came from a state with such records. It was less difficult to find information about the medical officers. They were licensed physicians before enlisting, so information about their medical schooling, their specialties, and their professional and home addresses was included in the 1918 edition of the *American Medical Directory*.

It is assumed that all of the enlistees of Field Hospital No. 33 chose to be in the Army Medical Department. Did having worked in a medical field upon enlistment aid in one's advancement? It was found that, among the 14 sergeants mentioned in Sergeant Brown's diary, the only pharmacists to became sergeants were Sergeant Brown and Sergeant Arthur Fisher. Although they did not become sergeants, Private Erwin Rubley and Private Marco Adragna were pharmacists before the war and continued in that profession afterwards. They did not advance beyond the rank of private first class. Not all of the soldiers of Field Hospital No. 33 were researched, so there may have been others that were of that profession.

Not including the six medical doctors researched, of the 28 enlisted men who were researched, only two other soldiers had worked previously in a medical field other than pharmacy. Sergeant Steven Lombard was an embalmer and continued in that field after discharge. Private John Biddle worked in a laboratory before the war, but what kind of laboratory we do not know. He did, however, work both before and after his Army service in a mental hospital as an attendant. Private Lawrence King chose medical-related work afterwards, and then only briefly. He worked for a government agency that was responsible for the return of the remains of soldiers who died overseas in World War I.

Where did the men enlist? A little bit of research revealed that recruiting offices were conveniently located near where enlistees lived. The offices were merely gathering and transferring points. Once they agreed to enlist, the men would be sent to a receiving station, where they would undergo a physical. If they passed, they would be accepted into service. Most enlistees from the Philadelphia area were sent to Fort Slocum, New York.[1] Other soldiers in Sergeant Brown's outfit from Central Pennsylvania went to the Columbus Barracks in Ohio, several hundred miles away from their homes.

Enlistees could choose which branch of the Army to join. A draftee did not have that choice. One could no longer enlist after December 17, 1917, however. All able men who were not in the service by that date and thus drafted would be assigned to whatever branch the Army choose.

Enlisting in the Medical Department was probably an attractive choice. A soldier in that field would be less likely to be ordered directly on the battlefield and subject to the onslaught of machine gun fire and the vicissitudes of trench warfare. They would not have to kill and maim but would help restore life. Soldiers in ambulance companies and aid stations, which were part of the Army Medical Department, worked very close to the front and would be directly in contact with enemy fire. A field hospital, which would normally be several miles from the battle, would be in less danger. It could still be susceptible to artillery and aerial bombing, however. In Field Hospital No. 33, Sergeant Brown's company, only one soldier out of about 140 died during the war. That was Fred P. Eberle, a wagoner, who died from pneumonia after the Armistice.[2]

One could not enlist after he received a notice from the draft board that he should appear for a physical examination. Sergeant Brown mentions his uneasiness that this could happen when he wrote to his parents the day he enlisted. That letter expressed his concern that he might be drafted before he was properly able to sign up. That letter appears in the introduction to the diary.

---

1. *Philadelphia Inquirer*, November 26, 1917, 2.
2. Christian Albert Bach and Henry Noble Hall, *The Fourth Division: Its Services and Achievements in the World War* (Country Life Publishers 1920), 358.

Appendix B

The Identification of Service Personnel as It Developed During World War I

Army service numbers, or serial numbers, were first issued to service personnel in February 1918. It had been found that the old method of maintaining personnel through rosters and muster rolls was too cumbersome for maintaining a huge army.

Enlisted men were assigned a six-digit number, while draftees were assigned a seven-digit number. The service numbers were first assigned on February 1, 1918. Officers were not given numbers because at that time there were relatively few officers. Eventually officers did receive serial numbers but not until after the war. Although the numbers of the enlisted men in Field Hospital No. 33 are close in sequence to one another, the only significance was that they were in the same company when the numbers were assigned.

Biographies of Selected Personnel Mentioned in Sergeant Brown's Diary

Arrowsmith, Private Ernest Henry

Service number: 571406

Ernest Arrowsmith was born in England on January 8, 1892, to James and Rachel (Lupton) Arrowsmith.[3] He came to the United States in 1901. His mother and his older brother John had previously immigrated in 1885. Apparently, his father had either died before then, or did not come to the United States.

In 1910 Ernest lived at 2400 Beale Avenue in Altoona, Pennsylvania, along with his brother, their mother, and their nine-year-old sister, Ethel Mae. Ernest had quit school after the eighth grade and was working as a laborer in a steam railroad shop.

On September 9, 1914, Ernest married Margaret Thomas of Oreminea, Pennsylvania. She was the daughter of John and Margaret Thomas. Ernest was 22 and Margaret was 16.[4]

On November 24, 1917, when he was living at 608 20th Street in Altoona, he enlisted at the Columbus Barracks in Ohio in the Medical Department. After enlistment he was sent to Fort Oglethorpe, Georgia, for

---

3. Pennsylvania World War I Veterans Service and Compensation Files, 1917–19.
4. Pennsylvania Marriages 1852–1968.

his basic training. Originally he was assigned to Field Hospital No. 34, but on December 1, 1917, he became attached to Field Hospital No. 33 at Camp Greene, North Carolina.[5]

The *Altoona Tribune* reported on November, 22, 1917, that Ernest had enlisted in the Army Aviation Service, but his service card stated otherwise.[6]

On the passenger list of the RMS *Melita*, which sailed from New York Harbor on May 27, 1918, Ernest's wife, Margaret, is listed as his next of kin. She was living at 412 20th Street in Altoona. The *Melita* arrived at Liverpool, England, on June 9. He arrived back to the United States at the port of Philadelphia aboard the SS *Minnesotan* from Brest, France, on August 3, 1919. He never advanced beyond the rank of private. While in France, Ernest, along with the rest of his company, participated in three campaigns: Aisne-Marne, Saint-Mihiel, and the Meuse-Argonne.

In 1920 Ernest and his family lived at 928½ 17th Street in Altoona. They had a daughter, Ethel, born about 1916. He was working as a blacksmith for a steam railroad.[7]

Ernest and Margaret had two other daughters and a son. These all died in infancy. According to the death certificate, one daughter who was born in July of 1917 died of malnutrition a little over three months later.[8]

In February of 1920, Margaret was badly burned when her dress caught fire from the stove she was using to keep warm. The child she was pregnant with lived briefly afterwards. Margaret died from complications 20 days later.

Margaret and the infant children were buried in the Oak Ridge Cemetery in Altoona.[9]

Ernest married Jennie Henry in Cumberland, Maryland, in 1929.[10]

In 1934, Earnest was awarded a veteran's compensation by the Commonwealth of Pennsylvania of $10 a month for 20 months.

In 1940 Ernest and his second wife, Jennie, rented their house at 1420 3rd Avenue in Altoona for $20 a month. Also living with them was Ernest's daughter, Ethel Mae, and her husband, John Henry. John was working as a mechanic's helper in a garage, and Ethel Mae was a salesgirl in a department store. Ernest worked as a blacksmith's helper in a railroad shop. His yearly income was $1,420.[11]

---

5. Pennsylvania World War I Veterans Service and Compensation Files, 1917–19.
6. *Altoona Tribune*, Altoona, Pennsylvania, November 22, 1917, 12.
7. 1920 U.S. Census, Altoona, Pennsylvania.
8. Pennsylvania Death Certificates, 1910–1967, for Ernest Arrowsmith.
9. https://www.findagrave.com/.
10. *Altoona Mirror*, July 6, 1970.
11. 1940 U.S. Census, Altoona, Pennsylvania.

He had worked as a blacksmith in the Juniata shop of the Pennsylvania Railroad for 49 years before he retired in 1956. He was a member of the VFW and the Methodist Church.[12]

Ernest died on July 4, 1970, after an extended illness at the Paoli Hospital in Paoli, Pennsylvania. He was 78 years old. He was survived by his wife; his daughter, Ethel Henry; two grandchildren; and three great-grandchildren. His second wife, Jennie Henry Arrowsmith, died in November of the same year. He was buried in the Geeseytown Cemetery in Frankstown, Pennsylvania, along with Jennie.[13]

* * * * *

Barkman, Private Frank Delost

Service number: 571407

Frank Barkman was born on October 15, 1896, in Ransomville, New York, to Frank A. and Mary Rosezella (Noyes) Barkman.[14]

In 1905 the family was living on Seaman Road in Niagara, New York. He had one older brother, James, born about 1891. His father was working as a farm laborer. Both of his parents were born in the United States.[15]

At age 14, young Frank appeared to have dropped out of school.[16] Frank's formal education ended after the eighth grade.[17]

While living in Oil City, Pennsylvania, on November 27, 1917, he enlisted in the army at Columbus Barracks, Ohio.[18] Like most of his fellow soldiers, he probably did his first Army training at Camp Greenleaf at Fort Oglethorpe, Georgia, before coming to Field Hospital No. 33 at Camp Greene, North Carolina.

While in the Army, Frank was diagnosed with tuberculosis sometime before March 15, 1918, according to Leland's diary entry of that date. But it was not until July 5, 1918, that he was sent to the U.S. Army General Hospital No. 18 in Waynesboro, North Carolina. That hospital was predominantly a hospital for tuberculosis patients.[19]

He was honorably discharged at Camp Wadsworth, Spartanburg, South Carolina, on March 15, 1919. He was reported to be 50 percent disabled

---

12. *Altoona Mirror*, July 6, 1970, 36.
13. https://www.findagrave.com/.
14. Ancestry member adrian_Barkman.
15. 1905 New York State Census, Niagara, New York.
16. 1920 U.S. Census, Hartland Township, Niagara County, New York.
17. 1940 U.S. Census, Celoron, Chautauqua County, New York.
18. Pennsylvania World War I Veterans Service and Compensation Files
19. https://history.amedd.army.mil/booksdocs/wwi/MilitaryHospitalsintheUS/chapter 26.HTM, 544–5.

at that time, presumably because of the lasting effects of tuberculosis.[20]

Frank was 22 when he married Emily Ada Potts in Charleston Township, North Carolina, on March 22, 1919.[21] This was just seven days after he was discharged from the hospital. Although one source states that Ada was born in Scotland, both the 1930 and 1940 U.S. Censuses show that she was born in North Carolina. Ada was the daughter of John T. Potts and A.M. Sheppards Potts.

He and Ada were living Alto, Tennessee, on June 25, 1921, when he applied for and was awarded the World War I Victory Medal for his service in the war even though he never served overseas.[22]

In 1920 they were still living at the same place as in 1905. His father was working as a laborer, doing odd jobs.

In 1930 Frank and Ada were living at 97 State Highway, in the 9th Civil District of Franklin County Tennessee. Frank did general farm work. By 1930, they had seven children: Frank Jr., age 10; James, eight; John, six; Austin, five; Ruth, almost three; and Carl, about a year old.[23]

They moved to Chautauqua, New York. In March of 1934, Frank applied for compensation as a veteran from the Commonwealth of Pennsylvania. It was approved, and he was awarded $10 a month for 16 months.[24]

In 1940 they still lived in Chautauqua. Frank at age 43 was unable to work, and Ada was keeping house. Their son William, 20, was working as a laborer in a furniture factory. He had completed the seventh grade. William earned a total of $154 for working only 14 weeks; James, 18, had finished one year of high school and was employed in road construction in a Civilian Conservation Corps camp. His earnings for 34 weeks of work was $252. John at 16 had completed the eighth grade, and Austin, 15, was in the eighth grade in school. The younger children—Ruth, 12; Carl, 10; and Mildred, 8—were all in school. All the children were born in Tennessee, except for William, who was born in North Carolina.[25]

In 1942, when Frank filled out his World War II draft registration card, he was living at 109 Chandler Street in Jamestown, New York. He was 5'7½" tall, weighed 164 pounds, and had blue eyes, brown hair, and a ruddy complexion. It was noted that he had a scar on his left cheek.[26]

Frank Delost Barkman died on November 22, 1955, in Busti, New

---

20. Pennsylvania World War I Veterans Service and Compensation Files.
21. North Carolina Marriage Records, Swain County, 1871–1958, for Frank Barkman.
22. Pennsylvania World War I Veterans Service and Compensation Files.
23. 1930 U.S. Census, Franklin County, Tennessee.
24. Pennsylvania World War I Veterans Service and Compensation Files.
25. 1940 U.S. Census, Celoron, Chautauqua County, New York.
26. World War II Draft Registration Cards, 1942.

York, of a heart attack while he was gathering Christmas decorations.[27] He was 59. He was buried in the Lakeview Cemetery in Jamestown, New York. He was a member of the American Legion and the Disabled American War Veterans.[28] He was nicknamed "Chum."

In 1946, while he was serving as a sailor in World War II, Frank and Ada's son Austin was killed in an accident at the U.S. Naval Air Station in Norfolk, Virginia. He was also interred in the Lakeview Cemetery.[29]

Ada, Frank's wife, died on April 16, 1966. She was buried alongside her husband. Also in the same cemetery are the graves of their son James Edward Barkman (1921–1969) and his wife, Elsie Bock Barkman (1923–1994).[30]

* * * * *

Biddle, Private John Young

Service number: 571408

John Young Biddle was born in Elkton, Maryland, on September 5, 1895,[31] to Cecil C. Biddle, a farmer, and his wife, Guila Young Biddle. He was one of seven children.

John's mother died in 1904, and his father died in 1910 when John was 14. The family was residing in Lancaster, Pennsylvania, with his eldest sister, Laura, and her husband, Harry Mullakin. Harry was a clerk at the courthouse in Lancaster.[32]

Three years later, John was working as an attendant in an insane asylum in Lancaster.[33]

In 1916 he was employed in Wilmington, Delaware, in a laboratory and living at 1123 W. 4th Street.

In May of 1917 he was an attendant at the Warren State Hospital for the Insane at North Warren, Pennsylvania. He was shown to be of medium height and build, with gray eyes and auburn hair.[34]

On September 28, 1917, while living at 18 Chester Street in Lancaster, Pennsylvania, he enlisted in the Medical Department of the Army at the Columbus Barracks in Ohio.[35]

---

27. New York State Death Index, 1852–1956.
28. *Post* (Jamestown, New York), November 23, 1955.
29. Virginia Death Records for Austin Paul Barkman.
30. Findagrave.com, Lakewood Cemetery, Lakewood, New York.
31. World War I Draft Registration Card, John Young Biddle.
32. 1910 U.S. Census, Lancaster, Pennsylvania.
33. Lancaster City Directory for 1913.
34. World War I Draft Registration Card, John Young Biddle.
35. *Lancaster New Era*, September 20, 1919, 10.

He was at the recruit camp of the Medical Officers Training Corps at Camp Greenleaf, Georgia, until November 17, 1917, when he became attached to Field Hospital No. 33 at Camp Greene, North Carolina.

After his training at Camp Greene was completed, he sailed on May 27, 1918, to Europe with his company on the RMS *Melita*. He returned to the United States on August 3, 1919, on the SS *Minnesotan*. He was discharged six days later at Camp Dix, New Jersey.[36] He was not wounded or disabled while in the service.

He served in the following campaigns, as did most of his fellow soldiers of Field Hospital No. 33: Aisne-Marne, Saint-Mihiel, and Meuse-Argonne, as well as in the Defensive Sector.

After his discharge from the Army, he returned as an attendant in the same hospital where he worked before the war: the Warren State Hospital for the Insane.[37]

Soon he married Sara Frances Wilson in Michigan.

By 1926, the Biddle family had moved to California, where he was working as a pipe fitter.

Unfortunately, John and four other workmen died as a result of an explosion at the Shell refinery at Dominguez, Carson City, California, on August 13, 1929.[38] He was 35 years old.

He was buried at the Roosevelt Memorial Park in Gardena, California. At graveside a bugler played "Taps," and he was saluted by riflemen from nearby Fort MacArthur. Also present were members of the local post of the Veterans of Foreign Wars who performed the last rites for their fallen comrade.

He left four children: Warren, 6; Gordon, 4; Albert, 2; and Charlotte, 4 months.

In 1936 his widow, Frances Biddle, applied and received a World War I veteran's compensation of $200 from the State of Pennsylvania. She was then living in Scott County, Iowa.[39] She died on January 10, 1969, in Oxnard, California.[40]

* * * * *

---

36. *Lancaster New Era*, September 20, 1919, 10.
37. 1920 U.S. Census.
38. Commonwealth of Pennsylvania Veteran's Compensation Application for John Y. Biddle.
39. Commonwealth of Pennsylvania Veteran's Compensation Application for John Y. Biddle.
40. California Death Index, 1940–1997; Clipping from an unknown newspaper posted by staciecl47 on Ancestry.com.

Bowman, Sergeant Jess Burdette

Service number: 571371

Jess Bowman was born on April 7, 1894, in Somerdale, Ohio, to Jess Bowman and Flora Geisinger.[41]

On September 13, 1913, when Jess was 19, he married Bertha Ellen Davy, daughter of James Davy and Olive Amanda Geisinger. Their marriage license showed only his mother's name.[42]

On June 14, 1914, Jess and Bertha Ellen had a son, James.

On July 4, 1917, Jess registered for the draft. He was working as a machinist for the Johnson Bronze Company in New Castle, Pennsylvania. He was married, yet his registration card showed that he had no dependents to support. He was described as being tall and slender with blue eyes and brown hair. He claimed that he had a crippled arm and was disabled.[43]

Jess Bowman enlisted in the Army at the Columbus Barracks, Columbus, Ohio, on September 25, 1917.

He received his preliminary training with the Medical Officers Training Corps at Fort Oglethorpe, Georgia, remaining there until November 11, 1917, when he joined Field Hospital No. 33 at Camp Greene, North Carolina. He was promoted to private first class on January 14, 1918, and he was promoted to sergeant about a month later.[44]

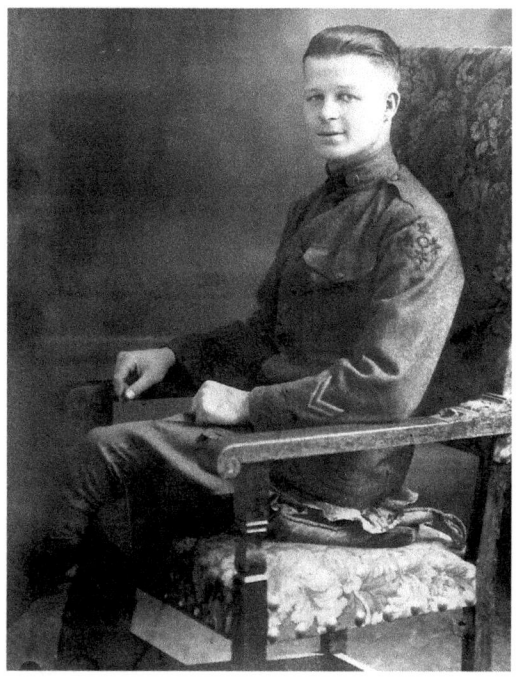

Sergeant Jess Bowman in Europe. He is showing his six-month overseas stripes on his left sleeve as well as the 4th Division shoulder patch (courtesy of Janice L. Bowman).

---

41. World War II Draft Registration for Jess B. Bowman.
42. Ohio County Marriages, Tuscarawas County, 1910–1915.
43. World War I Draft Registration Cards, 1917–1918, for Jess Burdette Bowman.
44. Ohio Military Men, 1917–1919.

The Personnel of Field Hospital No. 33

After his training at Camp Greene, he sailed from New York Harbor on May 27, 1918, on the RMS *Melita* to Europe with Field Hospital No. 33.[45] Sergeant Brown wrote what Bowman dictated, to a "girl" in the States. A small image of her appears in the September 25, 1918, entry of Brown's diary. It is unknown whether Bowman was writing to his wife or to another woman.

In France he participated in the following campaigns: Champagne-Marne, Aisne-Marne, Saint-Mihiel, Meuse-Argonne, and the Defensive Sector.[46]

On November 6, 1918, while he was in Europe with Field Hospital No. 33, Jess's wife, Bertha Ellen, died.[47]

Sergeant Bowman returned to the United States on the SS *Texan* from Brest, France. The *Texan* sailed on July 24, 1919, and arrived in Norfolk, Virginia, on August 6. He was no longer with Field Hospital No. 33 but with the 4th Division's Medical Mobile Degassing Unit. His next of kin was his mother Flora Rutledge of Midvale, Ohio.[48]

In January of 1920 he was one of two boarders at 207 East Ely Street in Alliance City, Ohio. At that time, he was working as a hammer man in a forge works.[49] His son, James William Bowman, who was about six years old, was living in Franklin Township, Ohio, with his maternal grandparents, James and Olive Davy.[50]

On August 5, 1922, Jess married Erma F. Wood. They had three sons: Robert Thomas (born 1924), Donald Charles (born 1926), and Gerald Lee (born 1935).[51]

In 1938, Jess's mother, Flora Geisinger Bowman, died.[52]

In 1940, Jess and his family were living on Haidet Road in Marlboro, Ohio. Their house (which they owned) was valued at $1,800. They had been at that address since 1935 and possibly before. Jess worked as a railroad conductor. Although employed for only 28 days during that last year, his income was $1,300. In the same household with Jess and his wife were their three sons: Robert, 15; Donald, 13; and Gerald, 5. It was noted that Erma had completed high school, while Jess had only finished eighth grade.[53]

---

45. U.S. Army Transport Service passenger lists, 1910–1939.
46. Ohio Military Men, 1917–1919.
47. Ancestry.com member jochannwr.
48. U.S. Army Transport Service passenger lists, 1910–1939.
49. 1920 U.S. Census, Alliance City, Ohio.
50. 1920 U.S. Census, Franklin Township, Ohio.
51. Ancestry.com member Jt31766.
52. Ancestry.com member Jt31766.
53. 1940 U.S. Census, Marlboro, Ohio.

In 1950, there was a record of a Jess Bowman being arrested for a misdemeanor and convicted of evading a taxi fare in Chattanooga County, Georgia. Instead of paying the $61.50 fine, he served 53 days of his two months sentence. The convicted Jess Bowman—born in 1894, 5'11" tall, 145 pounds, with blue eyes and dark brown hair, according to the Chattanooga County Jail's description[54]—bears resemblance to the Jess Burdette Bowman who registered for the World War II draft; the latter was 5'10" with blue eyes, brown hair, and a light complexion. On November 6, 1960, James William Bowman, the son of Jess and his first wife, Bertha Ellen Davy, died in Stark County, Ohio.[55]

On October 2, 1968, Jess Burdette Bowman died in New Smyrna Beach, Volusia, Florida. He had moved there from Ohio around 1961. He was a conductor with the Pennsylvania Railroad and a member of the Brotherhood of Railroad Trainmen. He was survived by his wife, Erma Bowman, and their three sons: Robert of Durand, Wisconsin; Donald, of Cuyahoga Falls, Ohio; and Gerald of North Canton, Ohio.[56] He was 74 years old.

In 1987, Jess's second wife, Erma Wood Bowman, died on October 5, 1987.

Erma and Jess are buried in the Alliance City Cemetery in Alliance, Ohio, along with their two infant children who had each lived less than a year.[57]

* * * * *

Cooper, Corporal Raymond Johnson

Service number: 571414

Raymond Cooper was born on October 19, 1896, in Lancaster, Pennsylvania, when his mother Carrie L. Cooper was 17. His father is unknown. Both of Raymond's parents were from Pennsylvania. Carrie was the daughter of Samuel and Etta Miller Cooper of Lancaster.[58]

Raymond's mother, Carrie, married Walter Tshudy in 1899. Neither Carrie nor Walter had been previously married.[59] Walter was an umbrella patcher in Lancaster, where the couple lived.

In 1907, during a Fourth of July celebration, Raymond was badly

---

54. Georgia Central Register of Convicts.
55. Ancestry.com member mmbowl1.
56. *Orlando Evening Star* (Orlando, Florida), October 4, 1968, 6.
57. Findagrave.com, Alliance City Cemetery, Alliance, Ohio, Jess B. Bowman.
58. 1900 U.S. Census, Lancaster, Pennsylvania.
59. Pennsylvania Marriages, 1852–1968, Lancaster County license #15930.

injured when a fire balloon sponge[60] fell suddenly, igniting his clothes and burning him on his neck, face, and shoulders.[61]

On June 19, 1917, when Raymond was living at 750 Queen Street, Lancaster, he enlisted in the Army at the Columbus Barracks, Ohio. He was originally assigned to the 54th Infantry at Camp Greenleaf until November 1, 1917, when he was attached to Field Hospital No. 33 at Camp Greene. He was promoted to corporal on May 6, 1918. On November 3, 1918, however, he was reduced to private for an unknown reason.[62]

When his outfit, Field Hospital No. 33, sailed from New York Harbor on May 27, 1918, on the RMS *Melita*, his next of kin was his mother, of Trenton, New Jersey. He arrived at Liverpool, England, on June 9, 1918.[63]

While with Field Hospital No. 33 Raymond served with his company during the campaigns of Aisne-Marne, Meuse-Argonne, and Saint-Mihiel.

After returning to the United States aboard the SS *Minnesotan* in 1919, he was discharged at Camp Dix, New Jersey, on August 6, 1919.[64] He then lived at 724 South Queen Street, Lancaster, with John Cooper, a relative; John's wife, Mary; and their daughter, Catharine. Raymond was working as a molder in a carbon steel company. John Cooper was a secretary at a cemetery.[65]

On December 31, 1920, Raymond married Marie Elizabeth Emig in Lancaster. She was the daughter of George and Elizabeth Emig. The Emigs were born in Pennsylvania of German ancestry.

In 1930 Raymond and Marie were living with her parents at 565 Christian Street, Lancaster. Raymond was working as a molder in a novelty factory. Marie's father, George, was a housepainter.

In 1934, Raymond applied for and received a veterans pension from the Commonwealth of Pennsylvania of $10 a month for 20 months.[66]

By 1940 Marie and Raymond were still living with her parents at the same address as in 1930. The Emigs owned their house, valued at $2,400. Everyone in the household had the same job they held in 1930.

Raymond's World War II draft registration card showed that he was 5'6" tall with a ruddy complexion, brown eyes, black hair, and a burn

---

60. A fire ballon sponge is a small hot-air balloon in which the heat necessary to propel the balloon skywards is provided by a lit sponge, often soaked in alcohol. The balloons are often made of paper and are therefore easily susceptible to catching on fire.
61. *Lancaster Intelligencer Journal*, July 5, 1907.
62. Pennsylvania World War I Veterans Service and Compensation Files, 1917–1919.
63. U.S. Army Transport passenger lists.
64. U.S. Army Transport passenger lists.
65. 1920 U.S. Census, Lancaster County, Pennsylvania.
66. Pennsylvania World War I Veterans Service and Compensation Files, 1917–1919.

scar on his throat. The scar was most likely from the accident when he was 10.[67]

On April 10, 1943, Raymond's stepfather, Walter Tshudy, was killed when he fell from a ladder.[68]

About a year later, Raymond's wife, Marie, died.[69]

Raymond Johnson Cooper died on November 7, 1944, at the Veterans Administration Hospital in Saratoga, New York. He was a member of the International Order of Fellows, the Knights of Malta, and the American Legion. He had been a molder at the Hubley Manufacturing Company in Lancaster, a company known for manufacturing cast-iron toys. He was 48 years old.

Raymond was buried next to his wife in the Greenwood Cemetery in Lancaster.[70]

* * * * *

Curran, Captain George Lally

George Lally Curran was born in North Adams, Massachusetts, on December 24, 1887, to Charles J. and Catherine Lally Curran.[71]

The elder Currans were both of Irish ancestry.[72] George was the third of seven children. George's father was a practicing physician. The family lived at 63 Eagle Street in North Adams.[73] In 1908, George's mother died.

George attended St. Joseph's School in North Adams and later went to the Northside Preparatory School in Williamstown, Massachusetts. Before he studied medicine and received his MD degree from New York University, he attended Holy Cross College in Worcester, Massachusetts.[74]

His father died in December of 1910 at age 49, just a few months after George joined his practice in North Adams.

On his World War I draft registration card of 1917, George was described as tall and stout, with brown eyes and brown hair.[75]

He was commissioned as a first lieutenant in the Medical Department on February 13, 1918, and called to active duty. At first, he was assigned the Walter Reed Hospital, but on July 31, 1918, he sailed from New York Harbor

---

67. World War II draft registration card for Raymond Johnson Cooper.
68. *Sunday News* (Lancaster, Pennsylvania), April 13, 1943, 24.
69. *Lancaster Intelligencer Journal*, April 10, 1944.
70. *Lancaster New Era*, November 8, 1944.
71. Massachusetts Birth Records, 1840–1915.
72. 1900 U.S. Census, North Adams, Massachusetts.
73. 1910 U.S. Census, North Adams, Massachusetts.
74. *North Adams Transcript*, June 29, June 30, July 2, July 3, and July 5, 1938.
75. World War I draft registration card, North Adams, Massachusetts.

aboard the RMS *Empress of Asia*. Listed as his next of kin was his eldest sister, Mary Curran.

He was assigned to Base Hospital No. 50 in August of 1918 near Mesves, France. This was the hospital in which 1st Sergeant Leland Brown was a patient from October 15, 1918 until January 12, 1919, when Brown returned to his outfit in Germany.

While at Base Hospital No. 50, Sergeant Brown worked with Lieutenant Curran doing patient reports and other office work for him. It is implied, from Leland's diary entries, that Lieutenant Curran kept him on after he recovered from being gassed because Curran needed him there.

After his work at Base Hospital No. 50, Curran was transferred to Base Hospital No. 103, which was near Dijon, France. While in France, he had been promoted to the rank of captain. The French government awarded Captain Curran a silver medal of honor for his "most enlightened and devoted care."[76]

Curran returned to the United States on the ship USS *Great Northern*, which arrived at Hoboken, New Jersey, on July 6, 1919.

Less than a month after his return to the States, George married Claire Elizabeth Russell in Chicago. She was the daughter of Charles Edward Russell, a lumberman of Seattle. Claire had been a Red Cross nurse stationed with Base Hospital No. 50, where they met. In his diary, Sergeant Brown mentions her in his January 9, 1919, entry: "I went to La Charite yesterday for Lieut. Curran. He has quite a case on Miss Russell, one of the nurses here. I bought some flowers for the Lieutenant and brought them back to the hospital."

After returning home to North Adams, he continued in his practice in conjunction with his brothers, Arthur and William, who were also practicing physicians. Together they converted the family home on Eagle Street into a medical center, which they named The Charles J. Curran Memorial Clinic to honor their father. The clinic included all the appurtenances of a modern hospital. There were operating rooms as well as a complete surgical theater and an X-ray laboratory.

George had limited his activity to obstetrical and gynecological work, while Arthur and William rounded out the practice. In 1923 Arthur left the clinic, followed by William in 1925. This required George to downsize the clinic.[77]

George and Claire had two sons, George Lally Jr. and Charles Edward Curran. Like his father, George Sr. died unexpectedly at a young age of a cerebral hemorrhage on June 30, 1938, at 50 years of age. He was buried at

---

76. *The National Cyclopedia of American Biography*, vol. 28, 852.
77. *The National Cyclopedia of American Biography*, vol. 28, 852.

the St. Joseph Cemetery in North Adams. Claire moved to Missouri to be closer to son Charles. There she died at the age of 87.

Both of their sons were Army veterans of World War II.

George was on the staff at the North Adams Hospital; a fellow of the American College of Surgeons; and a member of the American Medical Association, the American Legion, the Veterans of Foreign Wars, Knights of Columbus, Benevolent and Protective Order of Elks, and the Rotary Club of North Adams. He enjoyed hunting and the companionship of dogs.[78]

* * * * *

Daniel, Private First Class Guy Rogers

Service number: 571383

Guy Daniel was born on June 18, 1900, to William Frank and Angela Lilace (Rogers) Daniel in Columbus, Arkansas.[79] His father was from Arkansas of Georgia parents, while his mother was born in New Zealand to parents of English and Sicilian birth.[80] His father, William Frank Rogers, was a minister in the Nazarene faith, an evangelical Protestant religion.

In 1917 Guy enlisted in the Medical Department of the Army. He, like most if not all in the Medical Department, was first trained at Camp Greenleaf, Georgia, then further trained at Camp Greene, North Carolina, where he was attached to Field Hospital No. 33.

On January 16, 1918, Guy was promoted to private first class. About two weeks later, he was chosen for special training in administering ether and chloroform.

Like most of his fellow soldiers of Field Hospital No. 33, Guy was with his company when it participated in the following campaigns of the 4th Division in 1918: Aisne-Marne from July 18 to August 6, Saint-Mihiel from the September 12 to 16, and the Meuse-Argonne from September 25 until the Armistice on November 11, 1918. He then participated in the occupational duty in Germany.

When Sergeant Brown was gassed in France on September 30, 1918, Guy took care of him. In his diary, Brown wrote, "Daniel sent me to bed. That boy sure did look after me."

He and his company returned to the United States on the SS *Minnesotan* on August 2, 1919. The passenger list gives his sister Ruby as his next of

---

78. *The National Cyclopedia of American Biography*, vol. 28, 852.
79. Daniel Family Tree, Ancestry.com.
80. 1900 U.S. Census, Waldo, Arkansas.

kin. With both of his parents still living and older siblings, Ruby—11 years old—appears to have been an unusual choice.

By 1919, Guy's family had moved to 701 East 49th Street in Los Angeles. The 1920 U.S. Census showed that Guy was the oldest of the five Daniel children: He had three brothers—Wells, 19; Ira, 14; Edwin, 7—and a sister Ruby, age 12. Guy was unemployed.[81]

In 1930 Guy and his wife of six years, Clara Iris (Dickson) Daniel, were living on 649 South Burnside Avenue in Los Angeles. Guy was working as an investment sales manager. They rented their home for $55 a month.[82] They had only one child, June Iris Daniel, who was born on June 5, 1930.[83]

In 1935, while working as the advertising editor for the *Los Angeles Times*, Guy established a scheme to thwart fraudulent advertising by offering a $100 reward for the conviction of anyone using the "Business Opportunity" column to defraud. The scheme was successful in exposing a crime ring that stole furs and clothing.[84] He deployed a similar strategy when he was later employed by the *San Francisco Examiner*, increasing the reward to $250.[85]

On or about September 5, 1938, while living in San Francisco, Guy married Enid C. MacDonald.[86]

In 1940 Guy was working as a newspaper editor.[87] They both had completed high school.

In 1955 Guy and Enid were living at 172 Beach Road in San Rafael, California.

On April 1, 1959, Guy married Louise Hubbard Beattie in Marin, California. She was 48 years old.[88]

On July 5, 1972, after a long illness, Guy Daniel died while he was living in Vista, California. He was 71. He was survived by his wife, Louise; his daughter June St. John; and several grandchildren. He was a lieutenant commander in the Navy during World War II in charge of landing craft in the South Pacific on the assaults on Eniwetock and Kwajalein. He served in the Korean War as well. He was a member of the San Francisco Yachting Club and the San Francisco Advertising Club. He was buried in the Maple Grove Cemetery in Concord, Michigan.[89]

* * * * *

---

81. 1920 U.S. Census, Los Angeles, California.
82. 1930 U.S. Census, Los Angeles, California.
83. *San Diego Tribune*, October 8, 2017.
84. *Los Angeles Times*, February 28, 1935, 32.
85. *San Fransisco Examiner*, June 5, 1972, 56.
86. *Oakland Tribune*, September 5, 1938, 7.
87. 1940 U.S. Census, San Francisco, California.
88. California Marriage Index, 1949–1959.
89. *Times-Advocate* (Escondido, California), June 6, 1972, 25.

Delo, Private Carmen Chester

Service number: 571415

Carmen Delo was born on November 6, 1898, in Forest County, Pennsylvania, to John Adam Delo and his wife, Amelia Florence McDowell Delo. Both of Carmen's parents were born in Pennsylvania, as were his grandparents.

In 1910 the family was living in Green Township in Forest County, Pennsylvania. Carmen had four brothers and a sister. The two older boys, William and Albert, were working as laborers in a sawmill. His father was doing odd jobs. They rented their house.[90]

Carmen enlisted in the Army on December 29, 1917, at Fort Thomas, Kentucky, while he was living in Oil City, Pennsylvania.[91]

He probably did his preliminary training at the Officer's Reserve Training Camp at Camp Greenleaf, Fort Oglethorpe, Georgia, and his advanced medical training at Camp Greene, North Carolina.

Along with the most of his company of Field Hospital No. 33, he sailed to Europe on the RMS *Melita* on May 27, 1918.

Carmen participated in the following engagements in France while with Field Hospital No. 33: Aisne-Marne, Saint-Mihiel, and Meuse-Argonne. Although his service record states that he was not wounded while in the service, that record showed that he was attached to a casual company from September 20 to November 27, 1918, before returning back to Field Hospital No. 33. Perhaps he had been gassed or was sick.[92] For some unknown reason, if you were gassed in the Army, you were not considered to have been wounded. This was the case with Sergeant Brown.

He returned from Europe on July 3, 1919, on the SS *Minnesotan* from Brest, France, to Hoboken, New Jersey. He was discharged from the Army at Camp Dix, New Jersey, three days later.[93]

After his service, Carmen and his family lived at 2 Pump House Road in Oil City, Pennsylvania. The U.S. Census shows that he had five siblings: William, Albert, Hugh, Ina, and John. All the men worked in a machine shop as machinists except John, age 14. Their father was employed as a machine shop laborer, while Ina and the youngest son, John, were in school.[94]

---

90. 1910 U.S. Census, Forest County, Green Township, Pennsylvania.
91. Commonwealth of Pennsylvania Veterans Compensation Files, 1917–1919, for Carmen C. Delo.
92. Commonwealth of Pennsylvania Veterans Compensation Files, 1917–1919, for Carmen C. Delo.
93. U.S. Army Transport Service passenger lists, 1910–1935.
94. 1920 U.S. Census, Oil City, Pennsylvania.

By 1930 Carmen had married Cecelia. They had two sons—Donald J., age seven, and Wallace, age five—and a daughter Marion, age four. They rented their home in Oil City at 318 East 3rd Street for $24 a month. Carmen worked as a railroad mechanic.[95]

In October of 1944 the Delo family was residing at 315½ East 3rd Street in Oil City when he completed the Veteran's Compensation Application from the Commonwealth of Pennsylvania. That application showed that he was married to Celia Swartz Delo, and that he had minor children to support: Donald, Wallace, Marion, and Richard. He was awarded $190 from the Commonwealth.[96]

In 1940 the family was still at 315 ½ East 3rd Street, which they then rented for $20 per month. His income in 1940 was $450 per year, leaving them only $210 to spend on food, clothing, and whatever else the family would need. Their children were all living with them. They were all in school except for Richard, then six. Both Carmen and Cecilia went no further in their schooling than the eighth grade.

In 1955 Carmen and Cecilia were living at 1955 Park Avenue in Buffalo, New York. He worked as a machinist. In 1960 they moved to 36 Rodney Avenue in that city.[97]

After retiring from the Pennsylvania Railroad in Oil City, Carmen was employed for 25 years by Manzel Company of Buffalo, New York. He had three sons—Donald, Wallace, and Richard—and a daughter, Mrs. Oran (Marion) Boyd.[98] The Manzel Company manufactured machinery.

Carmen's obituary shows that he died in the Veteran's Hospital in Buffalo, New York, on July 9, 1972, and that he had lived in the Buffalo area for his last 25 years.[99]

He was buried in the Emlenton Cemetery in Venango County, Pennsylvania. It appears that his remains were moved or that the grave site was originally reported incorrectly. His grave is now in the St. Michael Catholic Cemetery in Fryburg, Clarion County, Pennsylvania. He is buried next to his wife, Cecilia M. Schwartz Delo, 1898-1984.[100]

* * * * *

---

95. 1930 U.S. Census, Oil City, Pennsylvania.
96. Commonwealth of Pennsylvania Veterans Compensation Files, 1917–1919, for Carmen C. Delo.
97. Buffalo New York City Directory for 1955 and 1960.
98. *Oil City Derrick* (Oil City, Pennsylvania), July 11, 1974, 16.
99. *The Oil City Derrick* (Oil City, Pennsylvania), July 10, 1974, 16.
100. Findagrave.com, St. Michaels Catholic Cemetery, Fryburg, Clarion County, Pennsylvania.

Dick, Lieutenant Walter

Walter Dick was born in Philadelphia, Pennsylvania, on January 22, 1889, to Francis Dick and Anne (Peebles). The Dicks had immigrated from Scotland three years earlier. Walter's father worked as a bleacher in a silk works. Walter had an older brother, John, as well as three younger siblings: Albert, Annie, and Florence. The family lived at 1945 Germantown Avenue in Philadelphia.[101]

Walter went to Central High School in Philadelphia and played on its basketball team. After high school he attended the Medico-Chirurgical College of Medicine in Philadelphia and graduated with an MD degree in 1913. The Medico-Chirurgical College was on the north side of Cherry Street between 17th and 18th streets. In 1916 it merged with the University of Pennsylvania Medical School.[102]

According to his medical school yearbook, "Dickey" worked one year during his summer vacation in a hotel in the Poconos as a bellhop and another summer as a conductor on a trolley car in Atlantic City. That same yearbook writer was not

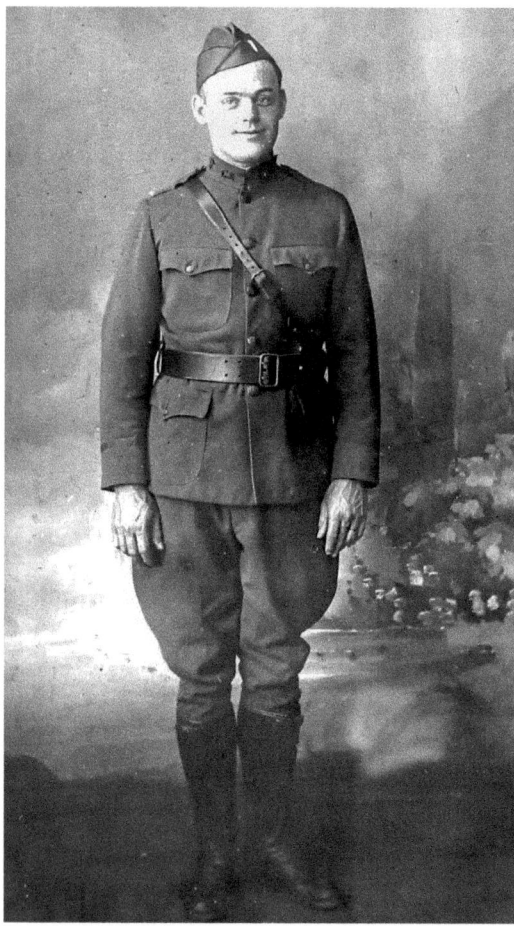

Lieutenant Walter Dick in uniform. This photograph was probably taken while in France while he was with Field Hospital No. 33 (University of Pennsylvania, University Archives and Record Center).

---

101. 1910 U.S. Census, Philadelphia, Pennsylvania.
102. Alumni Records of the University of Pennsylvania.

generous with him: "There must be some knowledge in him, little comes out" he quipped, and, "What Dick doesn't know about pathology would fill a book."

On his World War I draft registration card of June 5, 1917, he was shown to be of medium height and medium build, with gray eyes and brown hair. He was employed as the company physician for Shawmut Mining and Pittsburg and Shawmut Railroad in Ramseytown, Jefferson County, Pennsylvania. He claimed an exemption from the draft as he was "Doctoring Miners & Farmers & families."[103] Nevertheless, on October 10 of that year, while he was living in Ramseytown, he enlisted in the Army at Pittsburgh and received a commission as a 1st Lieutenant. He was 28 years old.[104]

He received his basic army medical training with the Medical Officers Training Corps at Camp Greenleaf, Georgia, until late December of that year, when he was attached to Field Hospital No. 33 at Camp Greene, North Carolina.

On April 30, 1918, Walter sailed to Europe on the USS *Finland* from Hoboken, New Jersey, along with his fellow medical officers from Field Hospital No. 33, Lieutenant Leighton Johnson and Captain Francis Fitzpatrick. They arrived in France about three weeks ahead of the others in the company and served as part of the Advanced School Detachment for the 4th Division, which established the training necessary for the company once it arrived in Europe.

Later in 1918, he served with the 39th Infantry and 12th Machine Gun Battalion, and then with the occupation forces of the A.E.F in Germany, until July 12, 1919—all of the 4th Division.

While he was in France he wrote a letter to his father. In that letter he described visiting his brother Albert, a private with the 95th Aero Squadron and his (Walter's) experiences with the Field Hospital:

33 Field Hosp. 4th Sanitary Train A.P.O. 746
Oct. 30, 1918

Dear Pop,

Well young fellow, how are you? You should be here helping to win the war instead of reading it in the papers.—but I guess you have done your share by sending your two sons over here. We are doing all we can to help Uncle Sam bring the Kaiser to his knees.

Mother and you and the girls would be proud if you could walk out on the aviation field and see machines flying all around and then see Albert working on one of the machines while the Lieutenant is waiting to take it up. Al knows his work and his officer likes him a lot. After the flier comes back from a flight with the boche he tells Al all about it and Al gets all excited and when I come around he tells me all about it. I

---

103. World War I draft registration card.
104. Pennsylvania World War I Veterans Compensation Files, 1917–1919.

believe Al's Lieut has made his last flight. He had downed many German planes but now I believe he is missing. Then let me take you to our Hospital where the ambulances are pouring in their wounded of all sorts among which are some boche wounded. Our boys have the proper spirit—they work in rain & mud with wet clothes & when they are seriously wounded they are still cheerful. We have missed many of the old faces from Colonels to the lowest private. The Hospital has been under fire. The ambulances shot up but our division has made a name for itself over here as one of the best. The men are tired but happy—they are doing all that the people back home expect of them and I believe more. They have been in the fight continuously and are making good. I'm feeling fine and I don't need anything. My fellow officers are all good fellows. Take good care of mother & Anna & Flora. Keep warm this winter. We'll be back soon.

Happy Xmas. Write me.

Walter Dick[105]

Walter returned to the United States on July 29, 1919, from the port of Brest, France, on the USS *Von Steuben*. He was then attached to the 12th Machine Gun Battalion.[106] He was honorably discharged four days later at Camp Dix, New Jersey.

On December 31, 1921, he married Mary Geist, the daughter of John and Louella Hopkins Geist. The wedding took place in the home of the bride on Jefferson Street in Brookville, Pennsylvania.[107] Mary's father was the president of the Brookville Title and Trust Company in Brookville. Mary's parents were living in Brookville, which was probably the reason why they settled there. Their home was on the corner of Church and Walnut streets. They had two children: Mary Ann, born in 1935, and Walter Jr., born in 1938.[108]

On his 1942 draft registration card, Walter was described as being 5'7", weighing 170 pounds, and having blue eyes, gray hair, and a light complexion.[109]

Walter Dick was the chief of staff at the Brookville Hospital; he had been living in Brookville for 31 years. He had been interested in athletics and coached some of the high school teams as well as being the team physician for some of the teams.

He was active in the Brookville American Legion, the Veterans of Foreign Wars, and the Kiwanis Club. He was also the president and a founder of the local county club, a Mason, and the director of the Chamber of Commerce in Brookville.[110]

---

105. Letter to home and photograph from the Pennsylvania Historical and Museum Commission via Ancestry.com.
106. U.S. Army Transport Service passenger lists, 1910–1939.
107. *The Brookville American* (Brookville, Pennsylvania), 1.
108. 1940 U.S. Census, Brookville, Pennsylvania.
109. World War II draft registration card.
110. *The Jefferson Democrat* (Brookville, Pennsylvania), February 8, 1951, 1.

Walter Dick suffered from arteriosclerosis. He died at his home of a heart attack on February 4, 1951, at age 62, and was buried in the Brookville Cemetery in Brookville, Pennsylvania.[111]

His wife, Mary Geist Dick, lived until August 25, 1999. She died in Brookville at 100 years of age.[112] She was buried next to her husband.[113]

* * * * *

Eberle, Wagoner Fred P.

Service number: 571385

Fred Eberle was born February 14, 1899,[114] to George L. and Marie (Nettie Gregg) Eberle.[115] His father, George, was an upholsterer. He had a sister, Marie, and a brother, George.[116]

Fred attended East High in Des Moines and grew up in the home of his cousin, David T. Davis. He enlisted in the Army on September 16, 1917, and was sent to Camp Logan at Denver, Colorado. From there he went to Camp Greenleaf at Fort Oglethorpe, Georgia, where he received his preliminary training. After Camp Greenleaf, he became attached to Field Hospital No. 33 at Camp Greene, North Carolina.

At some point in 1918, Private Eberle received the rank of wagoner. A wagoner at that time could either be a truck driver who hauled the field hospital's supplies as they moved from one location to the next or one who drove the hospital's animal-drawn supply wagons. The wagoner was also responsible for the care of the company's mules and horses.

On May 27, 1918, Fred, along with the rest of Field Hospital No. 33, sailed from New York Harbor on the RMS *Melita* to Europe. They landed at Liverpool, England, on June 7, 1918, and arrived in France four days later.

It is assumed that Wagoner Eberle was with his company when they participated in three major battles of World War I: Saint-Mihiel, Aisne-Marne, and the Meuse-Argonne campaigns.

Fred died of pneumonia in Saarburg, Germany, in December of 1918. His death date was reported to be either December 7 or December 17 of that month. His body was exhumed and returned to the United States on the U.S. Army transport *Antigone*, which sailed from Antwerp, Belgium,

---

111. Pennsylvania Death Certificates, 1906–1967.
112. *Punxsutawney Spirit*.
113. U.S. Find a Grave Index.
114. *Des Moines Register*, October 25, 1920, 1.
115. Iowa 1905 Census; 1900 U.S. Census Polk County, Iowa.
116. 1900 U.S. Census Polk County, Iowa.

on September 10, 1920, and arrived at Hoboken, New Jersey, 19 days later. His remains and those of others were grouped on the passenger list as "Remains of Overseas Dead."[117]

He was the only member of Field Hospital No. 33 to die in World War I.[118]

Hard maple trees were planted at his high school in Des Moines on April 30, 1919, to honor him along with 10 other students of East High who had lost their lives in World War I.[119]

He was buried in Des Moines with full military honors in the World War I Gold Star Memorial section of the Woodland Cemetery on October 24, 1920.[120] His gravestone is inscribed, "Fred P. Eberle, 1899–1918. Wagoner, 33rd F. Hosp. 4th Div."

* * * * *

Enwright, Private Philip Joseph

Service number: 571418

Philip Enwright was born on September 10, 1898, in Kenton, Kentucky, to Philip Enwright and Florence Eversman Enwright. His parents were both born in Kentucky, as were his grandparents. Philip's father was self-employed as a paper hanger. They lived on Pike Street in Covington City, Kentucky.

Philip had two brothers, George (born c. 1896) and Henry (born 1905), and three sisters: Gertrude (born 1901), Marie (born 1903), and Florence (born 1907).[121]

At some time in 1917, Phillip enlisted in the Medical Department of the Army. As most others of his company, he probably received his preliminary training with the Medical Officers Training Corps for several weeks at Camp Greenleaf, Georgia, before joining Field Hospital No. 33 at Camp Greene, North Carolina.

In the middle of December 1917, Philip, along with six other soldiers of Field Hospital No. 33, had contracted measles and was placed in a medical isolation detention camp. He was there until December 28.

In February of 1918, he went A.W.O.L. On March 1 of 1918, he returned and "was ready to take his medicine." He was placed in the guardhouse.

On May 7, 1918, Philip, along with Privates Walter Wigington and

---

117. U.S. Army Transport Service, Passenger List, 1910–1939, USAT *Antigone*.
118. Bach and Hall, *The Fourth Division*, 358.
119. *Des Moines Tribune*, April 25, 1919, 1.
120. *Des Moines Register*, October 25, 1920, 1.
121. 1910 U.S. Census, Covington City, Kentucky.

LeRoy Shearer, were reported A.W.O.L. and did not sail with their rest of Field Hospital No. 33 on May 27, 1918.[122]

At some point Enwright and Wigington either gave themselves up or were arrested and returned to active duty. Enwright and Wigington sailed to Europe on June 30, 1918, on the USS *Siboney* from Hoboken, New Jersey.[123] There was no further record of what happened to Shearer.

Philip married Mary Miller, probably in Gastonia, North Carolina, when she was 15. Mary was born in Tennessee to Noah and Harriet Miller.

After his discharge from the army, Philip lived with his wife's family at 610 Marietta Street in Gastonia. His 15-year-old wife and her sisters, Roe (14) and Minnie (17), all worked in a Gastonia cotton mill. Philip worked as a machinist, and the girls were spinners of cotton.[124]

Philip and Mary had two sons, Philip Joseph Jr., born on June 26, 1920, and Marshall Henry Enwright, born on August 9, 1921.[125]

Philip and Mary continued to live in Gastonia. In the 1950s and the '60s, Philip and Mary lived at 1115 Clouse Street there. He was employed as a salesman and a painter.[126]

Mary died on June 24, 1961, and Philip died on May 24, 1965, in Gastonia.[127] Philip was 66 years old. They are both buried in the Hollywood Cemetery in Gastonia, North Carolina, along with their son, Marshall Henry Enwright (1921–1981).[128]

* * * * *

Fisher, 1st Sergeant Arthur Raymond

Service number: 571373

Arthur Fisher was born in Saint Louis, Missouri, on April 22, 1894, to Maria (Mary) Heyens and John R. Fisher.[129] His father and mother were both born in Missouri. John's parents were from Germany and Switzerland. Maria's parents were from Germany.

In 1910, when Arthur was 15, he was apprenticed to a dentist. His father was an engineer in the stationery business. He had two sisters, Estelle (12) and Leona (three). Two other siblings of Arthur's had

---

122. Leland N. Brown diary.
123. U.S. Army Transport Service passenger lists, 1910–1939.
124. 1920 U.S. Census, Gastonia, North Carolina.
125. Ancestry.com, tmmillering.
126. City Directories for Gastonia, North Carolina, 1956, 1958, 1960.
127. Ancestry.com, tmmillering.
128. Findagrave.com, Hollywood Cemetery, Gastonia, North Carolina.
129. Missouri Birth Records, 1847–1910, for Arthur R. Fisher.

died before 1910. The family was residing at 2655 Iowa Avenue in Saint Louis.[130]

By 1917 Arthur was a pharmacist and a chemist living at 104 Maple Avenue in Jerseyville, Illinois. He was employed by the Jerseyville Ice & Coal Company there. He was described on his World War I draft registration card as having a medium build and height with blue eyes and brown hair.[131]

As there is no known record of Arthur attending a school of pharmacy, Arthur probably received his pharmaceutical training as an apprentice to a druggist, which at that time was a common practice.

Arthur enlisted in the Medical Department of the Army sometime in 1917. He probably completed his preliminary training at Camp Greenleaf, Fort Oglethorpe, Georgia, before taking his advanced training at Camp Greene, North Carolina. He was promoted to private first class on January 14, 1918, and about a month later he was promoted to sergeant.[132]

When he sailed from New York on the RMS *Melita* on May 17, 1918, from New York Harbor, his family was living at 403 Maple Avenue, Jerseyville, Illinois. He listed his father, John, as his next of kin. Along with most of his company, he arrived at Liverpool, England, on June 9, 1918.[133]

Arthur served in France with Field Hospital No. 33 during the following Army campaigns: Aisne-Marne, Saint-Mihiel, and Meuse-Argonne. He was promoted to sergeant first class sometime after September 23, 1918.

After the Armistice in November of 1918, his company was sent to Kaisersesch, Germany, where they were part of the A.E.F.'s occupation forces. He lived there in a house of the burgermeister with fellow sergeant Leland Brown. At some point when they were serving in Germany, Arthur and Leland traveled to Poitiers, France. There Leland attended lectures at the university. It is thought that Arthur also took classes at the university.[134]

Arthur was a bit of a cartoonist; three of his cartoons appear in Sergeant Brown's diary.

He returned to the United States on August 3, 1919, aboard the SS *Minnesotan*, which sailed from Brest, France, on July 23, 1919, and it arrived in Philadelphia along with most of his outfit. He was honorably discharged at Camp Dix, New Jersey, two days later. At that time, the Fisher family was living at 4131 Russell Avenue in Saint Louis.[135]

---

130. 1910 U.S. Census, Saint Louis, Missouri.
131. World War I draft registration card.
132. Leland N. Brown diary.
133. U.S. Army Transport Service passenger lists, 1910–1939.
134. Leland N. Brown diary.
135. U.S. Army Transport Service passenger lists, 1910–1939.

In 1920 he was living as a lodger at 3152 Grand Avenue in Saint Louis as a practicing druggist in a pharmacy.[136]

Later that same year he lived at 2653 Iowa Avenue in Saint Louis. His father was an engineer in the stationery business. He had two younger sisters, Estelle and Leona. His maternal grandmother, Elizabeth Heyens, was also living with them.[137] He was working as a clerk in the Grand Drug store in Saint Louis.[138]

In 1926, when Arthur was about 32 years old, he married Esther M. Fitzpatrick, the daughter of Thomas and Julia (Kaiser) Fitzpatrick.[139]

By 1930 Arthur was a drug salesman. He and Esther had two children, Donald J. (4) and Vera (almost 2). Their address was 5223 Bancroft Street, Saint Louis. Their rent was $37 a month and they had a radio.[140]

In 1940 the Fishers were living at 107 Allen Street in Chanute, Kansas. He reported that he was working 80 hours a week as the owner and manager of a retail drugstore. Esther was working as an unpaid assistant in their store for 60 hours a week.[141]

Arthur's 1942 draft card shows that they had moved to Freeburg, Saint Clair, Illinois. He was self-employed. That draft card also showed him being 5'9½" tall, weighing 167 pounds with blue eyes, brown hair, and a light complexion.[142]

On November 10, 1969, Arthur's wife, Esther Fitzpatrick Fisher, died.[143]

When Arthur died on December 29, 1970, he was living in Fenton, Missouri.[144] He was survived by his children, Donald Fisher and Vera Hill. He was buried next to his wife in the Mount Hope Mausoleum in Saint Louis, Missouri.[145] He was 76 years old.

* * * * *

Fitzpatrick, Major Francis Percival

Francis Fitzpatrick was born in Malden, Massachusetts, on June 18, 1887, to James and Theresa (Ronan) Fitzpatrick. Francis's father was from

---

136. Saint Louis, Missouri, City Directory for 1920.
137. 1920 U.S. Census.
138. Saint Louis, Missouri, City Directory for 1920.
139. Ancestry.com, Kenneth Robison.
140. 1930 U.S. Census.
141. 1940 U.S. Census.
142. World War II draft registration cards, 1942.
143. *Saint Louis Post Dispatch*, November 11, 1968, 18.
144. Social Security Death Index, Arthur R. Fisher.
145. Social Security Death Index, 1935–2014.

Ireland and worked in the United States as a laborer. Theresa was born in Nova Scotia,[146] Canada.[147]

Francis attended Georgetown University, graduating in 1909. His home address while he was an undergraduate there was 96 Pleasant Street, in Malden, Massachusetts.[148] He later attended the Georgetown University School of Medicine, where he received his MD degree in 1913.[149]

In 1916 in the Youngstown City Directory he is listed as a physician and surgeon. His office was at the Federal Building there. The family was residing on Lincoln Avenue at Phelps Street then.

On December 1, 1914, he married Mary O'Neil, the daughter of John S. O'Neil and Mary (Coyne) O'Neil. Mary was born in Ohio, but her parents were from Scotland and Northern Ireland.[150]

Francis and Mary had one son, James, who was born on May 26, 1917.[151]

On his World War I draft registration card of June 5, 1917, it was noted that he was tall, of a medium build, and had gray eyes and brown hair. He was living at 58 Nelson Avenue in Youngstown, Ohio.

Francis enlisted in the Army on August 17, 1917. He was assigned to the Medical Officers Training Corps at Fort Oglethorpe, Georgia, until December 8, 1917.[152] This is where he received his basic army training as a medical officer.

When Field Hospital No. 33 was formed on November 1, 1917, at Camp Greene, North Carolina, Lieutenant Fitzpatrick was appointed its commanding officer.[153]

At the age of 30, he served as a lieutenant in the Medical Corps in the Officers' Reserve Corps. He was promoted to captain on December 14, 1917, and subsequently to major on May 24, 1918.

On April 18, 1918, he sailed to France from Hoboken, New Jersey, on the USNT *Finland*. Francis, Lieutenant Leighton Johnson, and Lieutenant Walter Dick arrived in Europe ahead of their company on April 30. On the passenger list of the *Finland*, Francis's next of kin was Mary, his wife. She was living at 6401 Hough Street in Cleveland, Ohio.[154]

Francis served as the commanding officer of Field Hospital No. 33 with

---

146. 1930 U.S. Census.
147. Birth Records for the City of Malden, Massachusetts, 1887.
148. List of graduates of Georgetown University, 1909, 36.
149. *American Medical Directory*, 6th edition, 1918.
150. 1930 U.S. Census.
151. 1920 U.S. Census, Youngstown, Ohio.
152. Ohio Military Men, 1917–1918.
153. Leland N. Brown diary.
154. U.S. Army Transport Service lists, 1910–1939.

the American Expeditionary Forces at Aisne-Marne, Meuse-Argonne, and in the Defensive Sector, from April 30, 1918, to November 4, 1918, when he received an honorable discharge. Why he was discharged before the end of the war, which happened seven days later, one can only speculate. Perhaps he was wounded or had some other infirmity and could no longer serve. He was replaced in command of Field Hospital No. 33 by Major John Phillips.

In 1924 the Fitzpatrick family were living at 58 Wilson Avenue in Youngstown, Ohio.[155]

Their son James, their only child, died on December 16, 1925, at age eight.[156]

In 1930 the family was living at 94 Robinson Road, Campbell, Ohio. His wife's brother, John O'Neil, a railroad brakeman, was living with them. No children are shown on the 1930 U.S. Census.[157]

Francis died on January 23, 1937, in Campbell, Ohio, of complications of the heart. He was 49. He was buried in the Mt. Calvary Cemetery in Youngstown, Ohio.[158]

* * * * *

Hind, Sergeant Edward Wellyn, Jr.

Service number: 571377

Edward W. Hind Jr. was born on August 6, 1892, in Oakland, California, to Edward W. Hind Sr. and his wife, Charlotte A. Hind. In 1900 Edward Jr. was the eldest child and their only son. His sisters were Charlotte A., Violet G., and Dorothy M. Hind. All of the children were born in California except Dorothy, the youngest, who was born in Pennsylvania.

Edward Sr. had immigrated from England in 1880, and Charlotte came to the United States 11 years later. In 1900 the family owned their home on Chicago Avenue in Alameda, California. The elder Edward was working as stonecutter.[159]

Edward's schooling consisted of completing only the first year of high school.[160]

In or around 1912 the family moved to New Hampshire. Perhaps there was a better opportunity for Edward Sr. to find work in the stone carving business.

---

155. Youngstown, Ohio, City Directory 1924.
156. Ohio Death Records, 1908–1932.
157. 1930 U.S. Census.
158. Ohio Death Certificate for Francis P. Fitzpatrick.
159. 1900 U.S. Census, Alameda, California.
160. 1940 U.S. Census, Fitzwilliam, New Hampshire.

Edward Hind Jr. was of medium height and build, with blue eyes and brown hair when he registered for the draft on June 5, 1917. At that time, he was living in Greenfield, Massachusetts, and working as a machinist with the Bickford Machine Company there. The Bickford Company made tap making machinery.[161]

On July 5, 1917, Edward enlisted in the Army.[162] He was probably sent to Camp Greenleaf at Fort Oglethorpe before being sent to Camp Greene, North Carolina, for the advanced training that he needed for working in an Army field hospital. At Camp Greene he joined Field Hospital No. 33.[163]

Edward was appointed private first class on January 14, 1918,[164] and became a sergeant before May 26, 1918, when he sailed to Europe on the RMS *Melita*. On the ship's passenger list Edward's next of kin was his mother, Charlotte, who was living at Fitzwilliam Depot in New Hampshire.[165]

While at Camp Greene, on February 1, 1918, he was appointed the company mechanic. Sergeant Brown wrote in his diary that he was a good man and "knows all there is to know about autos."

He returned to Philadelphia on August 3, 1919, from Brest, France, on the SS *Minnesotan*. He was honorably discharged two days later at Camp Dix, New Jersey.

In 1920 the Hind family was living on Depot Road in Fitzwilliam. Edward Jr. was working as a machinist. His older sisters were employed: Violet as a hospital nurse and Rachel a telephone operator.

By that same year the Hinds had added three additional children: James (16); Desiree (8); and Llewellyn (5). Desiree and Llewellyn were both born in New Hampshire.[166]

On November 1, 1925, Edward married Birdie Elaine Wayland.[167] She was born in Canning, Nova Scotia, and immigrated to the United States in 1905. She was five years older than Edward and a divorcée. Edward, at the time of their marriage, was working as an electrician.[168]

In December 1925, Edward Sr. died. Edward Jr. and Birdie either moved into his parents' home on Depot Road in Fitzwilliam after his father's death or were already living there. In 1930 their house had a

---

161. World War I draft card for Edward Wellyn Hind.
162. U.S. Department of Veterans Affairs Death File, 1850–2010.
163. See image of Eddie Hind from the diary entry of March 5, 1918.
164. Leland N. Brown diary.
165. U.S. Army Transport Service passenger lists, 1910–1939.
166. 1920 U.S. Census, Fitzwilliam, New Hampshire.
167. U.S. Army Transport Service passenger lists, 1910–1939.
168. New Hampshire Marriage and Divorce Records, 1659–1947.

value of $1,300. Edward was working as a foreman in an electric company.[169]

In 1940, Edward and Birdie Hind were still in Fitzwilliam. Their home was now valued at $2,000. He was employed as a supervisor foreman in "Electricity."[170]

In 1942 Edward registered for the Second World War draft. At that time he was working at the Derry Electric Company in Easy Jaffrey, New Hampshire. He was described as being 5'7½" tall and weighing 150 pounds. Also on the draft card it was noted that he had blue eyes, brown hair, and a light complexion.[171]

Edward's wife, Birdie, died in 1970, and Edward died on September 15, 1972, in West Haven, Connecticut. He was 80. Edward and Birdie were buried in the Village Cemetery in Fitzwilliam. There is no evidence that they ever had children.

* * * * *

Hodsdon, Sergeant First Class Merle Eldon

Service number: 571368

Merle E. Hodsdon was born on May 30, 1895, in Roxbury, Maine, to Edgar Fairfield Hodsdon and Lula Della Noyes. Edgar and Lula were both born in Maine. Merle had four siblings: Irving, Abbie, Harold, and Guy. They lived at 614 Prospect Avenue in Oxford, Maine. Merle's father worked as a farm laborer.

Merle completed only the seventh grade.

He enlisted in the Army at Fort Slocum, New York, on July 8, 1914. In 1915, he served at the Sandy Hook Proving Grounds (Middletown Township, Monmouth County, New Jersey).

He was promoted to private first class on July 14, 1914. He was attached to the Post Hospital at Fort Screven, Georgia, until June 6, 1917, then to Fort Oglethorpe, Georgia, until July 1, 1917. From Fort Oglethorpe he was sent to several field hospitals until he joined Field Hospital No. 33 at Camp Greene. He was already a sergeant when Field Hospital No. 33 was formed on November 1, 1917. He was promoted to sergeant first class February 12, 1918, to succeed Sergeant Carlos Mena.

He sailed to Europe with the rest of his company on the RMS *Melita*

---

169. 1930 U.S. Census, Fitzwilliam, New Hampshire.
170. 1940 U.S. Census, Fitzwilliam, New Hampshire.
171. World War II draft registration cards, 1942. Men were subject for the draft until the day before their 45th birthday, but they were required to register until they were 65.

and shared his second class cabin with Sergeant Brown. He was seasick for the first eight days of the voyage.

While in France with his company, he was involved in the following campaigns: Aisne-Marne, Saint-Mihiel, and Meuse-Argonne. He would have been eligible of the Victory Medal with four clasps: the previous three campaigns and the additional clasp, the "Defensive Sector."

He returned to the United States on the SS *Minnesotan* from Brest, France, and arrived in Philadelphia on August 3, 1919. He shared a cabin on the *Minnesotan* with Sergeants Brown and Fisher.

After World War I he was stationed at Fort Dodge in Iowa. He had the rank of sergeant in the Provisional Regiment, 4th Division, Gary City, Calumet Township, Gary, Indiana.

He mustered out the Army on June 4, 1920.

After leaving the military he returned to Maine. In 1931–35, he lived in Portland, Maine, at 384 Cumberland Street, working as an electrician. In 1936 he appeared to be without employment and had moved to an apartment at 152 Spring Street in Portland.

In 1940, he was a patient at Pinellas Veterans Hospital in Florida. He died on June 23, 1977, in Andover, Maine, and is buried in the Woodlawn Cemetery in Andover. He never married. He was 82.

* * * * *

Johnson, 1st Lieutenant Leighton Foster

Leighton Johnson was born on November 30, 1890, in Hingham, Massachusetts, to Samuel F. and Dora A. (Belcher) Johnson. His father was a clergyman born in Ohio of Ohio-born parents. His mother was from Massachusetts of parents from that state. Additional children included Lottie, Meriam, and Herman.[172] The family was renting their home in Bourne, Massachusetts.

In 1915, Leighton graduated from the medical school of Boston University, and afterward he continued in his studies at Harvard Medical School.

On November 28, 1917, Leighton married Harriet Stanton Woodman in the District of Columbia.[173] Harriet, 19 years old, was born in Massachusetts, the daughter of William H. and Edith (Starrett) Woodman. Her father was a lawyer and was from Wisconsin. Her mother was from Canada.[174]

---

172. 1900 U.S. Census, Massachusetts.
173. District of Columbia, Compiled Marriage Index.
174. 1910 U.S. Census, Wakefield, Massachusetts.

When he registered for the World War I draft in 1917, Leighton was living at 869 Washington Avenue, Norwood, Massachusetts. He was shown to be of medium height and build, with light blue eyes and dark brown hair.[175]

At some time in 1917 he received his commission as a 1st lieutenant in the Army. He probably did his training at Camp Greenleaf at Fort Oglethorpe, Georgia, where most, if not all, of the officers of Field Hospital No. 33 gained their military training. He is first mentioned in Sergeant Brown's diary entry of February 22, 1918.

On April 30, 1918, Lieutenant Johnson sailed to Europe on the USS *Finland* from Hoboken, New Jersey, along with his fellow medical officers from Field Hospital No. 33, Captain Francis Fitzpatrick and Lieutenant Walter Dick. They were part of the Advanced School Detachment for the 4th Division, which prepared for the training necessary for the company once it arrived in Europe.

On June 17, 1918, five days after the company arrived in France, Lieutenant Johnson rejoined with Field Hospital No. 33.[176]

He returned to the United States aboard the SS *Rotterdam* from France on February 8, 1919, arriving at Hoboken, New Jersey, on February 17. On the passenger list his wife was shown as his next of kin. She was living on Mountain Avenue in Wakefield, Massachusetts. Lieutenant Johnson was listed as part of the Casual Officer's Detachment No. 45. This casual detachment contained "walking cases requiring no dressing."

Casual Officer's Detachment No. 45 consisted of transports from the Kerhuon Hospital Center in France. The hospital was four miles southeast from their port of embarkation at Brest, France, and about a mile and a half from the railroad. It was organized to be close to an embarking port to treat injured American soldiers before they returned to the United States.

There is an added note on the passenger list that the returnees would be sent to the Polyclinic Hospital in New York City. So perhaps Leighton had not fully recovered and required some medical treatment after his arrival.

In 1920 Leighton was in private practice and living at 31 Maple Street in Norwood, Massachusetts.[177]

In 1923 he and Harriet had a daughter, Judith Reynold Johnson, who died that same year.[178]

---

175. World War I draft registration card for Leighton F. Johnson.
176. Leland N. Brown diary.
177. 1920 U.S. Census, Massachusetts.
178. Findagrave.com for Leighton Foster Johnson, Pleasant Hill Cemetery, Wellfleet, Massachusetts.

By 1930 the family now included two sons: Leighton Jr., born about 1921, and David S., born about 1926. They were living at 78 Bond Street in Norwood, Massachusetts. In their household was a 27-year-old Black maid, Annie Lears. They owned their own home, which was valued at $20,000.[179]

From the '20s until 1952, Dr. Leighton's medical office was at 15 Bay State Road in Boston, a professional medical office building that he shared with dentists and other medical doctors. He lectured at Wellesley College and served as a consultant to hospitals in Natick, Fitchburg, Norwood, Nantucket, and Martha's Vineyard, all in Massachusetts.[180]

In April of 1941, when he registered for the World War II draft, the family had moved to 62 Ledgeways Street, Wellesley Hills, Norfolk, Massachusetts. It was noted that he had an appendix scar and that he was 5'9" tall with blond hair and a ruddy complexion.[181]

The Boston Guild for the Hard of Hearing relied upon him for consultations. The mission of the guild was to understand and address the problems of hearing loss.

Dr. Johnson was a Fellow of the American College of Surgeons and a member of the American Medical Association, the Algonquin Club of Boston, and the Boston Surgical Society.

For a time, he was head of the Ear, Nose and Throat Department at Massachusetts Memorial Hospital and the Boston University Medical School.

At the end of his life, he lived at Longwood Towers, Brookline, Massachusetts. Dr. Johnson died on July 21, 1953, at his summer home in Wellfleet, Massachusetts. He was 62.[182]

Leighton's wife, Harriet Woodman Johnson, died on January 10, 1987, at the age of 88. She is buried next to her husband in the Pleasant Hill Cemetery in Wellfleet, Massachusetts.[183]

Jongbloed, Sergeant Auke "Andrew"

Service number: 571375

Andrew Jongbloed was born on February 27, 1896, in Kubaard, the Netherlands, to Tjeerd and Janke van der Veen Jongbloed.[184]

---

179. 1930 U.S. Census, Massachusetts.
180. *Boston Globe*, July 22, 1953, 3.
181. World War II draft registration.
182. *Boston Globe*, July 22, 1953, 3.
183. Findagrave.com for Leighton Foster Johnson, Pleasant Hill Cemetery, Wellfleet, Massachusetts.
184. Petitions for Naturalization from the U.S. District Court for the Southern District of New York, 1897–1944 for Carolina Elizabeth Jongbloed.

In August of 1907, when he was 11, Andrew arrived in New York. He became an American citizen in 1918.[185]

On November 27, 1917, Andrew enlisted in the Medical Department of the U.S. Army.[186] It is assumed that he, as the rest of the company of the Field Hospital No. 33, received their preliminary training at Camp Greenleaf, Fort Oglethorpe, Georgia. He then came to Camp Greene, North Carolina, where he received his advanced field hospital training.

As with most of Field Hospital No. 33, Andrew sailed on the RMS *Melita* on May 27, 1918, from New York to Europe. He was no longer with Field Hospital No. 33, however, but attached the Headquarters of the Field Hospital Section of the Sanitary Train of the 4th Division. According to the passenger list of the *Melita*, his father, who was his next of kin, was living in Edmonton, Alberta, Canada.[187]

He returned to the United States on July 23, 1919, on the SS *Minnesotan* from Brest, France, which arrived at Philadelphia on August 3. His next of kin again was his father, who had immigrated to the United States.

In 1920 he was living with his parents and his brother John at 310 Hudson Street in Hoboken, New Jersey. Andrew was employed in the insurance business, and John was an

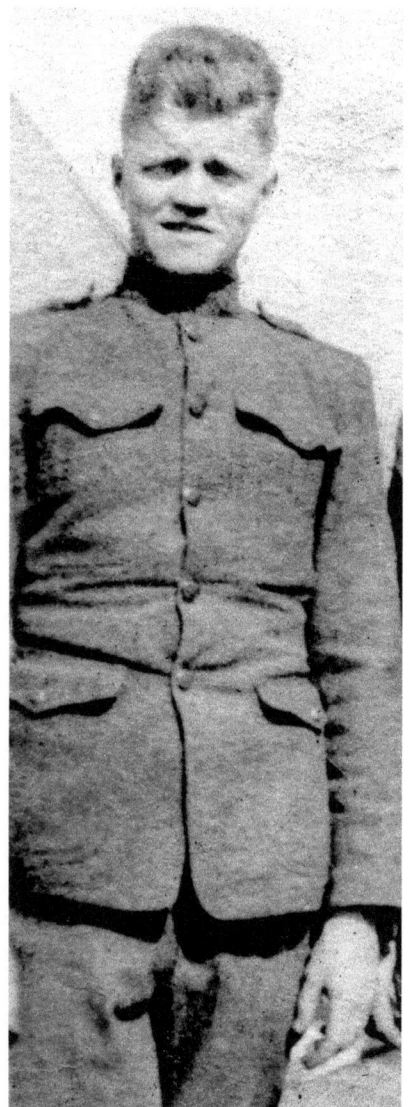

Sergeant Andrew Jongbloed at Camp Greene, North Carolina (photo album).

---

185. Petitions for Naturalization from the U.S. District Court for the Southern District of New York, 1897–1944 for Carolina Elizabeth Jongbloed.
186. Department of Veterans Affairs, Death File 1850–2010, Andrew Jongbloed.
187. U.S. Army Transport Service.

import broker. His father, Tjeerd, was a clergyman with the Dutch Christian Reformed Church.[188]

On November 29, 1922, Andrew married Carolina Elizabeth Hardenberg. She was the daughter of Jan Antonie and Carolina Elizabeth Vegel Hardenberg. Carolina was born on October 25, 1901, in Rotterdam, the Netherlands. Carolina and Andrew had two boys: Theodore, born in 1923, and Andrew, born in 1928. By 1926 they were living at 262 Page Avenue in Rutherford, New Jersey.

In 1930 Andrew was still working in the insurance business, but now they were living at 2 Van Eyk Court, in Lyndhurst, New Jersey. They rented their house for $45 a month.[189]

At some point on or before 1935, the Jongbloeds moved to an apartment at 62 Park Terrace West in New York City. Their rent in 1940 was $88 per month (about $1,600 in 2022 dollars). Their sons Theodore and Andrew were with them, as was Carolina's widowed mother, Carolina Hardenberg. Andrew was working as a real estate manager, possibly for the building in which they were living. Both Carolina and her mother had applied but had not yet received their U.S. citizenship. It was shown in the 1940 U.S. Census that Andrew had completed four years of high school, while his wife, Carolina, had only completed the eighth grade.[190]

In 1968 the Jongbloed family moved to St. Petersburg, Florida. Andrew died there on November 25, 1990, at age of 92. He was a member of the Veterans of World War I. He was survived by his wife and his two sons, eight grandchildren, and nine great-grandchildren. His wife died on September 26, 1993. Their two sons were veterans of World War II; Theodore was in the Marine Corps and Andrew Jr. was in the Army. Theodore was awarded the Purple Heart with one star for his service in World War II. A Purple Heart is given to a soldier who has been wounded in battle, while a Purple Heart with a star denotes that the recipient was wounded in two separate engagements.

Andrew's obituary implies that he was cremated. Both he and his wife have a grave site in the Bay Pines National Cemetery in Pinellas County, Florida. Their son, Theodore, and his wife, Blanche, have markers in the same cemetery.[191]

* * * * *

---

188. 1920 U.S. Census, Hoboken, New Jersey.
189. 1930 U.S. Census, Lyndhurst, New Jersey.
190. 1940 U.S. Census, New York City.
191. Findagrave.com, Bay Pine National Cemetery, Andrew Jongbloed.

King, Sergeant Lawrence D.

Service number: 571392

Lawrence King was born in Chesterhill, Ohio, on August 19, 1896, to Dorris King and his wife, Mary Sisk.[192]

In 1910 his father worked as a blacksmith in a coal mine. He had two brothers: Merrill W., who was born about 1890 and was employed as a yard clerk for a railroad company, and Cecil R., born about 1894. In 1910 the King family were renting a house at 149 Cherry Street in Trimble Township, Ohio.[193]

Lawrence enlisted in the Medical Department of the Army at the Columbus Barracks, Ohio, on September 16, 1917. He trained with the Medical Officers Training Corps at Camp Greenleaf, Georgia, before coming to Camp Greene, where he was attached to Field Hospital No. 33. On January 14, 1919, he was promoted to private first class and then to sergeant on May 1, 1918. In November of 1918, however, he was reduced to private first class. When he was honorably discharged at Camp Dix, New Jersey, in August of 1919, he had been reduced further to private for unknown reasons.[194]

While in France, he participated in the same campaigns as most of his fellow soldiers of Field Hospital No. 33: the Aisne-Marne, Saint-Mihiel, and Meuse-Argonne offensives.

In December of 1919, after he was discharged, Lawrence applied for a passport to travel to Great Britain, Belgium, France, Luxembourg, and Italy to serve as an assistant embalmer with the Graves Registration Service overseas. On that passport application he is described as being 5'9" tall with a high forehead, a straight nose, a medium mouth, a square chin, brown hair, a fair complexion, and an oval face.

The Graves Registration Service was established in August 1917 and was responsible for maintaining a burial recording system for deceased soldiers of World War I. Its mission included acquiring land in France for cemeteries and the return of soldiers' remains to the United States if requested by the next of kin.

On March 21, 1922, Lawrence returned to the United States after working for the Graves Registration Service on the SS *Cantigny* from Antwerp, Belgium, which arrived at Portland, Maine. The passenger list showed that he was single and living at 2053 Montrose Avenue, Chicago, Illinois,[195] the address of his parents.[196]

---

192. U.S. passport applications.
193. 1910 U.S. Census.
194. Ohio Soldiers of World War I, 1917–1918.
195. U.S. Atlantic Ports passenger lists, 1893–1959.
196. 1920 U.S. Census, Cook County, Chicago Ward, Illinois, for Dorris King.

In 1929, Lawrence married Susie Kessler, the daughter of Francis Kessler, a widower. In 1930 the Kings were living in the Kessler household in Divernon, Illinois, along with Susie's father and her three siblings. Lawrence and Susie's two brothers are all working on Susie's father's rented farm.[197]

In 1940, Lawrence and his wife, Susie, owned their own farm in Auburn, Illinois, that was valued at $9,500. He was working 70 hours a week, 52 weeks of the year. They had two children: Charles, age nine (born about 1931), and Doris Ann, age seven (born about 1933). The census of that year noted that both Susie and Lawrence had completed high school.[198]

On May 13, 1973, Susie died.

Lawrence died on September 15, 1985, in Auburn, Illinois, at the age of 89, and was buried with his wife in the Cumberland Sugar Creek Cemetery, Glenarm, Illinois.[199]

* * * * *

Lista, Private First Class Peter Pasquale

Service number: 571393

Peter Lista was born on March 12, 1899, in Delaware to Pasquale and Mary (Maria) Caruso Lista. Pasquale was a tailor. Both of his parents were born in Italy. His father was a naturalized citizen who had immigrated to the United States in 1886. The Listas lived at 617 Jefferson Street, Wilmington, Delaware. Peter is shown on the 1900 census as Pasquale. He had one sibling, Antonio, born in October of 1895.[200]

By 1910 Peter (Pasquale Jr.) had two other siblings: Nancy, age nine, and Louise, age four. They were living at 210 West 7th Street in Wilmington, where they rented their home.[201] In 1913 his sister Katherine was born.

Peter received an eighth grade education. On June 23, 1917, at age 18, he enlisted in the Army. He most likely took his preliminary Army training at Camp Greenleaf, Fort Oglethorpe, Georgia, before coming to Field Hospital No. 33 at Camp Greene.

He is mentioned several times in Sergeant Brown's diary. While in the Army he acquired the nickname of "Dodo." He played on the company's baseball team and performed in skits in towns the company visited while

---

197. 1930 U.S. Census, Sagamon County, Illinois.
198. 1940 U.S. Census, Auburn, Sagamon County, Illinois.
199. U.S. Social Security Death Index; Findagrave.com, Cumberland Sugar Creek Cemetery Illinois, Lawrence D. King.
200. 1900 U.S. Census, Wilmington, Delaware.
201. 1910 U.S. Census, Wilmington, Delaware.

at Camp Greene. He was promoted to private first class on January 16, 1918.

He traveled to Europe with his company on the RMS *Melita* from New York on May 27 and arrived at Liverpool, England, on July 7, 1918. During the war, his company was involved in the following campaigns: Aisne-Marne, Saint-Mihiel, and Meuse-Argonne. He would have been eligible for the Victory Medal with four clasps denoting the three campaigns in which Field Hospital No. 33 was involved. In addition, the "Defensive Sector" clasp was awarded for general defense service, not involving a specific battle.

After serving with Field Hospital No. 33 in France and Germany, he returned to the United States on August 3, 1919, from Brest, France, to Philadelphia aboard the SS *Minnesotan*, as did most of his company. Peter was honorably discharged at Camp Dix, New Jersey, after his return.

After World War I, Peter lived with his family in Wilmington and worked as a telegraph messenger.[202]

In 1927 he married Mary Elizabeth Matthews in Philadelphia.[203] Mary was born in South Wales, Great Britain.

By 1940 the Listas had two sons: Peter, age 11, and Edwin, nine. They owned their own home at 547 Cypress Street, in Yeadon, Pennsylvania, a suburb of Philadelphia. It was valued at $7,250. He worked at the Warwick Hotel in Philadelphia as the superintendent of services. The Warwick was one of the premier hotels in the city at that time. His yearly income in 1940 was $1,500, and he was working 60 hours a week.[204]

Evidently, he took his work at the Warwick Hotel very seriously. The following was reported in 1950 in the *Philadelphia Inquirer*:

> Apparently there's no such word as "impossible" in the vocabulary of Peter Lista, the Warwick's travel man. He was a bit stymied during the holiday, however, when a Mr. Executive of Sun Oil wanted plane reservations at the last moment. Peter dashed to the airport, and had his own "sit down" strike 'til he got what he wanted.[205]

His World War II draft registration card of 1942 noted that he was 5'2" tall, weighed 170 pounds, and had a ruddy complexion, black hair, and brown eyes. His name on that registration was Peter Pasquale Lista.

In the early 1950s the Listas kept a summer cottage near Stroudsburg, Pennsylvania.[206]

---

202. 1920 U.S. Census, Wilmington, Delaware.
203. Pennsylvania Marriage Index
204. 1940 U.S. Census.
205. *Philadelphia Inquirer*, April 16, 1950.
206. *The Pocono Record*, June 6, 1953, 25.

Peter was living in Yeadon on February 19, 1965, when he died of a heart attack at Fitzgerald Mercy Hospital in Darby, Pennsylvania. He was 65. He was buried at Valley Forge Gardens, King of Prussia, Pennsylvania.[207] Peter's wife, Mary Matthews Lista, died on March 5, 1972.[208]

* * * * *

Lombard, Sergeant First Class Steven Sherwood

Service number: 571376

Steven Lombard was born on February 14, 1893, in Addison, Michigan, to Edward A. and Mary Janette (Nettie) Marshall Lombard. Steven had two siblings: a sister, Neita, born in August of 1891, and a brother, Leon, born in 1894. His father was a general farmer on a farm that they owned mortgage-free. They were living in Wheatland Township in Michigan. Everyone in the family was born in Michigan except Steven's grandparents, who were born in New York.[209]

In 1910 the family was living on the same farm in Wheatland as in 1900. Steven and Leon were attending school.[210]

In June of 1917 Steven was living in Baltimore, Maryland. He was working as an embalmer for Charles F. Evans & Son of that city. His draft registration card noted that he had brown eyes and dark brown hair with a medium build and a medium height. He had previously been in the U.S. Navy as a hospital apprentice for four years.[211]

Sometime in 1917, Steven enlisted in the Medical Corps of the Army. That he chose the Medical Corps was not surprising, considering his medical background in the Navy. He, as other members of his company, trained with the Medical Officers Training Corps at Camp Greenleaf, Fort Oglethorpe, Georgia. When that was completed, he went to Camp Greene, North Carolina, where he continued his training with Field Hospital No. 33.

He received his first promotion on January 4, 1918, when he was appointed private first class. On February 15 of that same year, he was appointed sergeant. He was again quickly promoted to sergeant first class.[212]

On May 27, 1918, he sailed with the rest of Field Hospital No. 33 to

---

207. Pennsylvania Death Certificates, 1906–1967.
208. *Philadelphia Inquirer*, March 7, 1972, 31.
209. 1900 U.S. Census, Wheatland Township, Michigan.
210. 1910 U.S. Census, Wheatland Township, Michigan.
211. World War I draft registration card, Steven Lombard.
212. Leland N. Brown diary.

Europe aboard the RMS *Melita*. On that voyage he shared a second class cabin with first sergeants Merle Hodsdon and Leland Brown.

On December 16, 1918, he returned to the United States about six months before the rest of his company. He was then part of the sick and wounded contingent of Base Hospital No. 33. Evidently, he had been under medical treatment and was sent to the United States six months before other soldiers of his company.[213] He sailed from Liverpool, England, on December 8, 1918, on the USNT *Leviathan* and arrived at Hoboken eight days later. His next of kin was his father, Edward A. Lombard of Hanford, California. After landing at Hoboken, he was sent to a facility—cryptically noted on the passenger list as "D. H. #2"—for further treatment.

On March 10, 1920, Steven married Velma V. Wickland, age 22. Wilma was born in North Dakota of Swedish parents.

In 1930 Velma and Steven were living at 1629 Truxton Avenue in Bakersfield, California. There they rented their home for $100 a month. Steven continued in the undertaker business.[214]

Velma had sued in Los Angeles for divorce in October of 1931. The divorce wasn't granted until September of 1935.

In 1940 Steven lived at 2303 Rio Linda Boulevard in North Sacramento, California. In the same household was Ernest and Ruth Baugh, his gardener and housekeeper. Steven was working on his own account as an undertaker.[215]

In 1941 Steven married Rachel Riggs in Sacramento, California. She was about 39 years old, and he was 48. Rachel was a widow. At that time he was living at 521 South Gate Road in North Sacramento. His undertaking business was at 110 W. El Camino Avenue there.[216]

About 1946 Steven married Lavinia Parkin, a divorcée. Lavinia had previously been married and had had a child from that marriage.[217]

He died on March 30, 1957, at age 67, and was interred at the East Lawn Memorial Park in Sacramento.

His third wife, Lavinia, died on October 3, 1993, and was buried next to Steven. Lavinia was 86.

There was no record showing that Steven ever had children.

* * * * *

---

213. U.S. Army Transport Service passenger lists, 1910–1935.
214. 1930 U.S. Census, Bakersfield, California.
215. 1940 U.S. Census, North Sacramento, California.
216. World War II draft registration cards, Steven Sherwood Lombard.
217. Marriage records of Steven Sherwood Lombard were furnished by Vivian Lumbard on Ancestry.com.

Appendix B

Mannas, Private Charles Joseph

Service number: 3049884

Charles Mannas was born to Joseph H. and Flora R. Mannas on September 8, 1896, in Shippenville, Pennsylvania. Joseph was a farmer and owned his own home. Charles was one of 11 children. His parents were born in Pennsylvania and were of German and Irish descent.

Charles was drafted into the Army at Sapulpa, Oklahoma, on September 4, 1918. He was one of only 14 soldiers of Field Hospital No. 33 who were a draftees out of a total of 125 (not including officers). He was then living in Kiefer, Oklahoma, and working for the Chestnut and Smith Gasoline Company in Kiefer. He was described as being of a medium height and slender, with light blue eyes and light brown hair.

He was part of the Camp Greenleaf Georgia Replacement Unit No. 65 that sailed on October 19, 1918, from New York on the USS *Walmer Castle* to Europe. This was about a month before the Armistice, and he was not shown to have been in any military engagements.

Although he is not mentioned in Sergeant Brown's diary, he was with Field Hospital No. 33 until July 22, 1919, when he returned to the United States at Hoboken, New Jersey, on the SS *America* from Brest, France. In the passenger list of the *America*, he was listed with the Convalescent Detachment No. 369 of Brest, France. In that detachment he was grouped with the "walking patients requiring no dressings—class 'B.'"

Since he was with a convalescent detachment, he probably went to a hospital or other facility to recuperate after he returned. Because he wasn't discharged until two months later on September 24, the implication is that he was recovering from some ailment or wound before he was released from the Army. He was honorably discharged at Camp Pike, Arkansas. He was not promoted while he was in the service.[218]

On November 24, 1924, Charles was married to Linda Christina Olbert. Linda was born in Colorado to George and Anna Olbert, who had immigrated from Germany in the 1880s. George Olbert was a liquor dealer.[219]

Charles and Linda had at least four children: Robert, Earl, Donald, and Leroy. Leroy died in 1933 of pneumonia at four months of age.

In 1942 Charles was self-employed in a typewriter and adding machine business based at his residence at 236 Jefferson Street in Butler,

---

218. Pennsylvania World War I Veterans Service and Compensation Files, 1917–1919, Charles Mannas.
219. 1910 U.S. Census, 15th Precinct, La Plata County, Colorado.

Pennsylvania. It was noted that he was 5'6" tall, weighed 130 pounds, and had blue eyes, brown hair, and a light complexion.[220]

In June of 1969, Charles died at age 72 while living in Rockville, Maryland. He was buried in the Gate of Heaven Cemetery in Silver Springs, Maryland. His wife, Linda, died in 1998 and was buried beside him.

* * * * *

McDonnell, Private Thomas Francis

Service number: 571430

Thomas McDonnell was born on January 3, 1899, in Altoona, Pennsylvania, to James Patrick and Margaret (MaGowan) McDonnell.[221] Both of his parents were born in the United States.

In 1910 the McDonnell family was living at 1911 Sixth Avenue in Altoona. Thomas is shown as Francis McDonnell on the census. At that time, his parents had been married for 13 years. James was 50 and Margaret was 44. They have had five children, all living in 1910. The oldest was Paul, 12 (born about 1898). Their father was steadily employed as a molder in a railroad foundry. A molder is a person who prepares a mold for casting, usually that of iron.[222]

Thomas had completed two years of high school when he enlisted at Columbus Barracks, Ohio, on November 23, 1917, with his Altoona friend, Joseph Monahan.

At first he was at the recruit camp of the Medical Officers Training Corps at Camp Greenleaf, Georgia. He then became attached to Field Hospital No. 33 at Camp Greene, North Carolina.

In December 1918 while at Camp Greene, he was sent to a detention camp, there having contracted measles.[223]

He served overseas with Field Hospital No. 33, sailing on the RMS *Melita* from New York Harbor May 27, 1918, and landing at Liverpool, England, on June 9.

He was with Field Hospital No. 33 throughout his service overseas and until discharge. He and most of the members of that outfit participated in the following battles: Aisne-Marne, St. Mihiel, and Meuse-Argonne.

He was promoted to private first class on November 3, 1918; to corporal

---

220. World War II draft registration card.
221. Pennsylvania World War I Veterans Service and Compensation Files, 1917–1919, for Thomas Francis McDonnell.
222. 1910 U.S. Census, Altoona, Pennsylvania.
223. Leland N. Brown diary.

on November 16, 1918; and to sergeant on November 24, 1918. He was reduced to a private on May 1, 1919, while he was in Germany as part of the occupation forces of the 4th Division.[224] It is unknown why he was demoted.

He returned on the SS *Minnesotan*, which sailed from Brest, France, on July 23, 1919, arriving in Philadelphia on August 3 of that year. He was discharged three days later at Camp Dix, New Jersey.

He was not wounded while he was in the service.[225]

He was eligible for the Victory Medal with the following clasps: Aisne-Marne, Saint-Mihie, Meuse-Argonne, and the Defensive Sector.

In 1920 his family was still living at the same address as they were in 1910, which was mortgage-free. Thomas's father, James, was working as a soft iron molder for the railroad. Both of his mother's parents were from Ireland. All the children were unmarried.

Thomas's brother, Paul, age 22, was a pipe fitter for a steam railroad, Thomas, 21, was working as a machinist helper. Both Paul and Thomas were probably working for the Pennsylvania Railroad. He had two sisters: Sarah, age 16, and Catherine, age 13.

In 1930 the family was living in a house they owned, valued at $7,000. Living with them were his father, James, 61, and his single sisters: Sarah E., age 27, and Catherine, 24. James was still working as a molder for Pennsylvania Railroad. Thomas was working for the railroad as a boilermaker. Sarah was unemployed, and Catherine was a secretary in an electric power company.

In 1934 Thomas was awarded a World War veteran compensation of $200 by the State of Pennsylvania.

In 1940 the family was still together, living at the same address as in 1910. The value of their house had shrunk to $3,200, presumably because of deflation caused by the Depression. Thomas was still with his father, 80, and his two single sisters: Sarah E. and Catherine M. McDonnell. The 1940 census showed that Thomas had dropped out of high school after two years, but his sisters had completed all four years.

In 1939, Thomas worked 48 hours a week as a boilermaker in a "steam railroad shop." Sarah was unemployed, and Catherine was employed working 40-hour weeks as a secretary in a "light company." Thomas's salary was $1,000 a year, and Sarah's was $1,200. All three children were single.

Thomas's 1942 draft registration card showed that the siblings still lived at 1911 6th Avenue, where they had been since 1910 or before. He was

---

224. Pennsylvania World War I Veterans Service and Compensation Files, 1917–1919, for Thomas Francis McDonnell.
225. Pennsylvania World War I Veterans Service and Compensation Files, 1917–1919, for Thomas Francis McDonnell.

The Personnel of Field Hospital No. 33

working for the Pennsylvania Railroad at its 2nd Street Altoona Works. His next of kin was his father, James P. McDonnell, who was at the same address. Thomas was 6'1" tall, weighed 195 pounds, and had gray eyes, brown hair, and a ruddy complexion.[226]

In April of 1945, when James, Thomas's father, was 85, he died. James's obituary mentions that his daughter Catharine served as a staff sergeant in the Woman's Army Corps during World War ll.[227]

It appears that neither Thomas nor his two sisters ever married.

Thomas died on September 4, 1961, of complications of hypertensive heart disease after a short illness. He was buried in the Calvary Cemetery, in Altoona, Pennsylvania.[228]

He was a member of the Sacred Heart Catholic Church and Holy Name Society, the World War I Veterans, and the Veterans of Foreign Wars. He had worked as a railroad car repairman for 40 years with the Pennsylvania Railroad before his retirement.[229]

* * * * *

Monahan, Corporal Joseph Gerard

Service number: 571433

Joseph Monahan was born on August 26, 1899, in Altoona, Pennsylvania[230] to Thomas J. and Sarah Ellen (O'Connell) Monahan. In 1900 he was the youngest of seven living children. Everyone in his extended family had been born in Pennsylvania, except for his Irish-born maternal grandmother. Joseph's siblings, ages 11, 8, and 6, were attending school. They lived at 56 Eighth Avenue in Altoona.

His father was working as a locomotive engineer. His oldest brother, John, then 18, was an apprentice machinist. At that time, Altoona was the site of the largest railroad repair shops and manufacturing factories in the world, owned and operated by the Pennsylvania Railroad.

In 1900 they had a servant living with them, Sarah McTamany, a 58-year-old widow.[231]

---

226. World War II draft registration for Thomas McDonnell.
227. *Altoona Tribune*, April 11, 1945, 10.
228. Pennsylvania Death Certificates, 1906–1967, for Thomas Francis McDowell; Findagrave.com, Calvary Cemetery, Altoona, Pennsylvania, Thomas McDonnell.
229. *Altoona Mirror*, September 5, 1961, 23.
230. Pennsylvania World War I Veterans Service and Compensation Files, 1917–1919, for Joseph G. Monahan.
231. 1900 U.S. Census, Altoona, Pennsylvania.

The 1910 U.S. Census showed that while his mother had given birth to 15 children, by 1910 only eight survived.

His father, Thomas, worked as a railroad engineer, and three of his brothers are working for the railroad, either as a shop hand, a machinist, or a fireman. His older sister, Marie, was teaching music. Joseph, who would have been only about 10, was not listed with the rest of the family. The Monahans owned their house at 1917 Eighth Avenue in Altoona mortgage-free.[232]

Joseph enlisted at the Columbus Barracks, Ohio, on November 23, 1917, along with his Altoona buddy Thomas McDonnell. They both chose the Medical Department of the Army and were together throughout their enlistment. The local newspaper reported the following:

> Joseph G. Monahan, of 1917 Eight avenue, enlisted in the hospital corps ambulance department yesterday. He was a junior apprentice at Altoona machine shops, a well known athlete and a member of the De Neri and Altoona Cubs basketball teams. He departed last evening for Ft. Slocum N.Y.[233]

They did not enlist at Fort Slocum but at the Columbus Barracks in Ohio. Also enlisting at the same time for the medical department from Altoona was Earnest Arrowsmith and Harry N. Zeigler. Arrowsmith, like Monahan and McDonnell, served with Field Hospital No. 33. Zeigler, however, did not.

Joseph's residence when he enlisted was 1917 8th Avenue, Altoona, Pennsylvania. His next of kin was his mother, Sarah E. Monahan. Joseph had completed only two years of high school.[234]

He served overseas with Field Hospital No. 33, sailing from New York Harbor on May 27, 1918, on the RMS *Melita* arriving at Liverpool, England, on June 9.

He was with Field Hospital No. 33 throughout the time that he was in the service. Along with most of the members of that outfit, he saw service in the following battles: Aisne-Marne, Saint-Mihiel, and Meuse-Argonne.

He was promoted to private first class on November 3, 1918, and to corporal on November 26, 1918.[235]

He returned on the SS *Minnesotan*, which sailed from Brest, France, on July 23, 1919, and arrived in Philadelphia on August 3. He was discharged three days later at Camp Dix, New Jersey.

---

232. 1910 U.S. Census, Altoona, Pennsylvania.
233. *Altoona Tribune*, November 22, 1917, 12.
234. 1940 U.S. Census, Altoona, Pennsylvania.
235. Pennsylvania World War I Veterans Service and Compensation Files, 1917–1919, for Joseph G. Monahan.

The Personnel of Field Hospital No. 33   195

He was not wounded while he was in service.[236]

On August 9, 1919, the local newspaper, the *Altoona Tribune*, reported his return and that of his buddy Thomas McDonnell from the Army:

> Corporal Joseph Monahan and Thomas F. McDonnell, who returned to Altoona on Thursday [August 7], saw plenty of exciting service in France. While attached to field hospital 33 they went through Chateau Thierry, St. Mihiel, Belleau Wood and Argonne drives as stretcher bearers and field ambulance workers. Corporal Monahan is the son Mrs. S.E. Monahan of 1917 Eighth Avenue, while O'Donnell [sic] is the son of Mr. and Mrs A. McDonnell, of 1915 Sixth avenue. They enlisted together in 1917 and remained together throughout their period of service. After the Armistice, they were members of the army of occupation. They received their discharge from Camp Dix, N.J.[237]

His father, at 70, was no longer working. Joseph was again employed for the railroad as a machinist apprentice. His younger brother Herbert was driving a truck, while his other two brothers were working as machinists for a railroad, presumably the Pennsylvania Railroad.

In November 1920 Joseph's father passed away, and his mother, Sarah, became the head of the family. They were still living in the 8th Street property, which they valued at $3,000.

His brother Herbert lived there too, working as a truck driver for a dye works.[238]

Joseph married Helena Gertrude Hoelzle on June 26, 1929. Helena was born to Elizabetha (Wolf) and Joseph Hoelzle. The Hoelzles were from Germany.

In 1934 Joseph and Helena were living at 341 Lotz Avenue in Altoona with their two minor children, Patricia and Bernard. Joseph applied for a World War I veteran's compensation from the state of Pennsylvania and was awarded $200 for his military service.[239]

Joseph worked 30 40-hour weeks in 1940 as a repairman in a Pennsylvania Railroad railroad car shop. His yearly income was only $450. A neighbor who worked 40 weeks at what appears to be the same job received $1,000 for the year. They were renting their home at 341 Lotz Avenue for $15 a month. They had three children: Patricia, eight; Bernard, six; and Thomas, one.

When he filled out his World War II draft card in 1942, they were still living at the same address. He was working at the Pennsylvania Railroad's

---

236. Pennsylvania World War I Veterans Service and Compensation Files, 1917–1919, for Joseph G. Monahan.
237. *Altoona Tribune*, August 9, 1919, 13.
238. 1930 U.S. Census, Altoona, Pennsylvania.
239. Pennsylvania World War I Veterans Service and Compensation Files, 1917–1919, for Joseph G. Monahan.

Car Department on 12th Street in Altoona. He was described as being 5'9" tall and weighing 160 pounds with brown eyes, black hair, and a ruddy complexion.[240]

He was a member of St. John's Catholic Church in Lakemont, Pennsylvania, and the Catholic Knights of St. George.[241]

When Joseph died on February 19, 1979, he was residing at 202 North Pine Street in Lakemont, Pennsylvania.[242] He was 79. Lakemont is about four miles south of Altoona. He was buried at the St. Mary's Cemetery in Altoona.[243] His wife, Helena, died in 1985. She was buried beside him.

Mullaney, Private James Joseph

Service number: 571394

James Joseph Mullaney was born in Worcester, Massachusetts, on September 27, 1887, to Alice L. McGrath Mullaney and Thomas Francis Mullaney.[244] James's parents were from Ireland.

James married Mary Elizabeth Monaghan of Boston on June 6, 1906, in Worcester. He was 19 years of age and working as a teamster. Mary was 18.

By the summer of 1917, James had spent one year as a private with the Field Artillery of the Massachusetts Militia.[245] At that time he was employed as a gardener in his father's business. On June 5 of that year he registered for the draft. That registration showed him living at 52 Dewey Street, Worcester, Massachusetts. His draft card described him as being of average height and slender, with brown eyes and dark brown hair.

Private James Mullaney at Camp Greene, North Carolina (photo album).

---

240. World War II draft registration card for Joseph G. Monahan; 1940 U.S. Census, Altoona, Pennsylvania.
241. *Altoona Mirror*, February 19, 1979, 34.
242. *Altoona Mirror*, February 19, 1979, 34.
243. Pennsylvania Veteran's Burial Card, 1777–2012, for Joseph G. Monahan.
244. Massachusetts Marriage Records, 1840–1915.
245. U.S. World War I Draft Registration Cards, 1917–1918.

He enlisted in the Army Medical Department at Worcester, Massachusetts, on July 27, 1917. Perhaps he chose to enlist rather than risk being drafted. If he were drafted, he might be chosen by the Army to be in artillery due to his previous experience with the Massachusetts Militia.

At Camp Greene, North Carolina, where James was receiving his advanced training, he was mentioned five times in Leland's diary as being either A.W.O.L. or under arrest. Despite all of his transgressions, on January 18, 1918, he was promoted to private first class, and by May of 1918, when his company sailed to France, he had reached the rank of corporal. Yet he was listed as a private when he returned from France.

He was evidently diagnosed with tuberculosis while abroad, which delayed his return.

He was to sail on the SS *Aeolus* from Brest, France, on July 17, 1919, but his name on that list was crossed off. He was grouped with Tuberculosis Cases Class "C."

He arrived in Brooklyn aboard the USS *Ryndam* from Brest, France, on August 4, 1919. He was part of the Convalescent Detachment No. 385 and grouped with other Tuberculosis Patients Class "A." His mother, Alice Mullaney, was listed as his next of kin. She was living at 105 Fairmont Avenue, Worcester, Massachusetts.[246]

In 1920, he, his wife, Mary, and their two children were living in Winthrop, Massachusetts, with Mary's parents, Joseph and Mary Monaghan. In the same household were four of Mary's siblings, ranging in age from 35 to 20. James and Mary's two children were with them as well: Augustas, age 13, and Paul, nine. James is shown as being in "vocational training." Only Mary's two brothers and sisters were employed. Her father was not.

Sometime in 1921, the family moved to San Pedro, California, presumably for James's health. In various city directories he is shown as a clerk or working in the photography business.

For various terms, James was a patient at the Sawtelle Veterans Home in what is now Los Angeles. He was there for about three weeks in 1927 and for three months in 1928. His last visit was in January of 1929.[247]

In 1930 his family was residing at 1226 12th Street, San Pedro, California. Besides his wife, there was their 19-year-old son, Paul, an auto mechanic. James, unemployed, was probably in poor health and unable to work.[248]

James died in California on September 25, 1931, two days before his 44th birthday. His address was 1026 West 12th Street, San Pedro, California.

---

246. U.S. Army Transport Service passenger lists, 1910–1939.
247. U.S. National Homes for Disabled Volunteer Soldiers, 1866–1938.
248. 1930 U.S. Census, San Pedro, California.

In 1932, a grave marker was requested from the Office of Veterans Affairs by his wife, Mary. It was placed on his grave in the St. Peter's Cemetery in Worcester, Massachusetts.[249]

* * * * *

Paquette, Private Allen William

Service number: 571435

Allen William Paquette was born in Detroit, Michigan, on July 22, 1894, to William Paquette and Charolette Graham. His father, William, was born in Canada and his mother in Michigan.[250]

In 1910 Allen was living with his younger brother and their widowed mother. Allen, 15, was out of school and working in a railroad office as a bookkeeper.[251] By 1911 his brother, Albert, was also no longer in school and working. Presumably both Albert and Allen had quit school to help with the household expenses. The family was living at 171 Brainard Street in Detroit. Their mother was listed as Charolette Whitman, a widow.[252]

In 1915 the family moved to 129 Ledyard Street in Detroit. Allen was working in the printing business.[253]

When he registered for the draft on June 5, 1917, he claimed a deferment since he was supporting his mother. His draft card showed him as a sheet metal worker at the Cadillac Motor Company. He was of a medium height and build with blue eyes and brown hair.[254]

At some point during 1917,

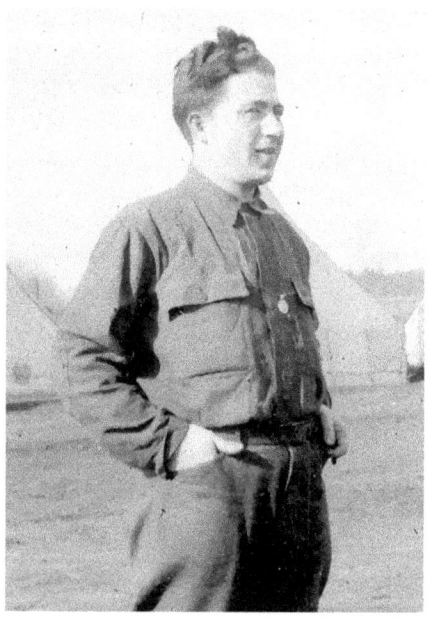

Private Allen Paquette at Camp Greene, North Carolina (photo album).

---

249. U.S. Headstone Applications for Military Veterans, 1925–1963.
250. 1900 U.S. Census, Detroit, Michigan.
251. 1910 U.S. Census, Detroit, Michigan.
252. 1910 U.S. Census, Detroit, Michigan.
253. Detroit City Directories for 1910, 1911, 1915.
254. World War I draft registration card for Allen Paquette.

Allen enlisted in the Army and was sent to Fort Oglethorpe, Georgia, for his basic training and then assigned to Field Hospital No. 33 at Camp Greene, North Carolina.

On April 22, 1918, a little more than a month before his unit shipped overseas, Allen married Edna L. Meyers of Culver, Indiana.[255]

The passenger list of the RMS *Melita* sailing from New York Harbor on May 27, 1918, shows his wife Edna listed as his next of kin. She was living in Culver. The *Melita* arrived at Liverpool, England, on June 9. He returned to the United States at the port of Philadelphia aboard the SS *Minnesotan* from Brest, France, on August 3, 1919.[256]

In 1920 he lived at 176 20th Street, Detroit, with his wife, mother, brother, and two boarders. Allen was working in a sheet metal factory, while Edna was employed as a stenographer in a hospital.[257]

By 1930 Edna and Allen had moved to 9012 Madison Avenue, Los Angeles. He was employed as a postal clerk, and Edna was a clerk in a veterans bureau. They owned their own home and had a radio.[258]

In 1940 their address was 819 Cypress Street in Glendale, California. Their house was valued at $5,500. His salary as a clearing office clerk at the post office was $2,100 per year. Their daughter, Anita, was three.[259]

By 1959 Allen had been promoted as the superintendent of the post office in Glassell Park Station (California). That postal station had a staff of 49 employees.

Allen Paquette died in Glendale, California, on March 15, 1967, at age 67.[260]

Phillips, Major John Charles

John Phillips Jr. was born on November 5, 1876, to a long-established Boston family.[261] He was the first-born child of John C. Phillips Sr. and Anna (Tucker) Phillips. Their younger children included William, born 1878; Anna F., born 1879; Martha R., born 1882; and Madelyn.

In 1880 the Phillips family lived at 111 Berkeley Street in Boston. His father, John Sr., was an East Indian Importer. Living with the family

---

255. Wayne County Marriage Records 1887–1925.
256. U.S. Army Transport Service lists.
257. 1920 U.S. Census, Detroit, Michigan.
258. 1930 U.S. Census, Los Angeles, California.
259. 1940 U.S. Census, Glendale, California.
260. *Los Angeles Times*, June 26, 1959, 148.
261. Findagrave for John Charles Phillips, https://www.findagrave.com/memorial/125867589/john-charles-phillips.

in 1880 were eight servants, who were from Nova Scotia, Scotland, and Ireland.[262]

John's parents and his grandparents were all from Massachusetts, except for his mother's father, who was from New Hampshire.[263] The Phillips family dated back to the 1700s in Massachusetts. His great grandfather, also named John Phillips, was the first mayor of Boston.

John attended Milton Academy in Milton, Massachusetts. He graduated from Harvard University in 1899 with a BA degree and received his MD degree from the Harvard Medical School in 1904.

On January 11, 1908, John married Eleanor Hayden Hyde of Bath, Maine. She was the daughter of Thomas W. and Annie (Hayden) Hyde.[264] Eleanor's father was born in Italy, and her mother was from Maine.[265] John and Eleanor had two sons and two daughters.

In 1915, before the United States was directly involved in the war with Germany, a volunteer group of medical personnel from Harvard University was organized to provide assistance to the British Expeditionary Force in Europe. John Phillips was part of a contingent—30 men and 38 women—of doctors, dentists, and nurses. They arrived on the *Noordam* in November of 1915 and saw their first patients on December 15 of that year at Camiers, France. They treated more than 1,400 patients over the next three months.[266]

During his service, John was given the rank of an honorary lieutenant in the British Army.

After the Harvard unit was demobilized from the British Army, he returned to America and joined the Medical Department of the American Expeditionary Forces, advancing in rank to major. He succeeded Major Francis Fitzpatrick as commander of Field Hospital No. 33 when Fitzpatrick, for some reason, was honorably discharged seven days before the end of the war.

After the war ended and Field Hospital No. 33 completed its occupational duty in Germany, Major Phillips sailed to the United States on the SS *President Grant* from Brest, France, and arrived at Boston on July 11, 1919. On the passenger list of that ship, he was shown as part of the Le Mans Provisional Battalion No. 237 of casuals. He was released to Boston, while most of the soldiers on the same ship were sent to Camp

---

262. Findagrave for John Charles Phillips.
263. 1880 U.S. Census, Boston, Massachusetts.
264. Massachusetts Marriage Records 1840–1950.
265. 1930 U.S. Census, Wenham, Massachusetts.
266. "David Cheever and the Second Harvard Unit," Center for the History of Medicine at Countway Library, https://collections.countway.harvard.edu/onview/exhibits/show/noble-work-for-a-worthy-end/harvard-surgical-unit/david-cheever-second-harvard.

Devens, Massachusetts. His wife and children were then living in Wenham, Massachusetts.[267]

After the war he served as the house surgeon for two years at the Boston City Hospital. Phillips then left his practice as a medical doctor and entered deeply into the study of wildlife. He traveled the globe to study and collect specimens of bird and mammal species for placement in natural history museums. He authored more than 200 papers and other publications in genetic studies of wild animals as well as their protection and their relation to the environment. His four-volume work, *A Natural History of the Ducks*, was considered the best in that field.

In 1930 John and his family were living at 77 Mount Vernon Street in Boston. Their house was valued at $45,000 ($730,000 in 2022 dollars). Their six servants included a cook, three maids, and a trained nurse. The Phillips children were John C. Jr., age 21; Madeline, age 17: Eleanor, age 15; and Arthur, 9. All the children were attending school.[268]

John gave large tracts of land in Boxford, Wenham, and Rockport, Massachusetts, for wildlife preservation. He was associate curator of the Harvard Museum of Comparative Zoology and president of the board of trustees of Peabody Museum and on the board of many other conservation organizations. He was also an associate curator at the Peabody Museum at Harvard and the president of the Massachusetts Fish and Game Association.

In 1946, The Division of Wildlife Research and Management occupied a former Civilian Conservation Corps camp in Upton, Massachusetts, and named it the John C. Phillips Research Lab in his honor.[269]

John's brother, William, had a distinguished diplomatic career including serving twice as the under secretary of state and the ambassador to Italy and other countries. His sister, Martha, married Andrew J. Peters, who served in the U.S. Congress and was also at one time the mayor of Boston.

The Phillips Wildlife Research Laboratory of the Division of Fisheries and Game was named for him. His grandson of the same name was later appointed commissioner of the Massachusetts Department of Fisheries, Wildlife and Recreational Vehicles.

John Phillips died of a heart attack on November 15, 1938, while on a hunting trip near Dover, New Hampshire.[270] His brother, William, arrived

---

267. U.S. Army Transport Service passenger lists, 1910–1939.
268. 1930 U.S. Census, Boston, Massachusetts.
269. The CCC (Civilian Conservation Corps) was a public work relief program that operated from 1933 to 1942 in the United States to help the young unemployed find work during the Great Depression.
270. *Boston Globe*, November 15, 1938, 15.

in New York on the *Queen Mary* and flew to Boston just in time for John's funeral.[271]

He was buried in the North Beverly Cemetery in Beverly, Massachusetts. He was 62 years old.[272]

* * * * *

Pitcairn, Captain Edward Alexander

Edward Pitcairn as born on March 15, 1886, in Derry, Pennsylvania, to Edward Pitcairn and his wife, Eleanor Jane ("Jennie") Fulton. His father was born in Ohio. His grandparents had come from Scotland. His mother, Jennie E. (as shown on the 1900 U.S. Census), was born in Pennsylvania, as were her parents. In 1900 his parents had been married 26 years and had four other children besides Edward. His father was employed as a train master. They were living at 832 Rebecca Avenue in a house that they owned mortgage-free. The house was located in what was known then as the Wilkinsburg Ward of Allegheny County, which probably later became incorporated into the city of Pittsburgh.[273]

Edward attended East Liberty High School in Pittsburgh before matriculating at Penn State College (now Penn State University), where he majored in mining. He was a member of the Phi Kappa Sigma fraternity.

After college, he enrolled in the Hahnemann Medical College in Philadelphia, graduating there in 1912. He was called into active service on June 13, 1917, as a 1st Lieutenant in the Medical Corps.

He sailed to Europe aboard the *Caserta* from Hoboken, New Jersey, on May 10, 1918. His next of kin was his wife, Alice Hammond Pitcairn, living at 624 Clyde Street, Pittsburgh.[274]

Edward served overseas until February 17, 1919. He was attached to the Evacuation Hospitals No. 5 and No. 6 of the 1st Division in Europe in the following campaigns: Séry-Magneval, Château-Thierry, Villers-Cotterêts, Ville-sur-Cousances, and La Veuve. He was promoted to captain on December 24, 1917.[275]

Although he is shown attached to the Provisional Field Hospital G on November 1, 1917 (later Field Hospital No. 33), he probably was transferred to Camp Crane in Allentown, Pennsylvania, where his services were

---

271. *Boston Globe*, November 17, 1938, 12.
272. Find a Grave Index, 1600–.
273. 1910 U.S. Census, Allegheny County, Wilkinsburg Ward, Pennsylvania.
274. U.S. Army Transport Service passenger lists, 1910–1939, *Castera*.
275. Pennsylvania World War I Veterans Service and Compensation Files, 1917–1919, Edward Alexander Pitcairn.

needed in the training of the ambulance service. This was before he was shipped overseas.

He sailed on the SS *Rotterdam* from Brest, France, on February 8, 1919, and arrived in the United States, at Hoboken, New Jersey, on February 17, 1919. He was discharged at Camp Upton, New York, on March 4, 1919.

In 1918, even though he was in Europe at the time, his residence was listed at 806 Rebecca Avenue, Wilkinsburg, Pennsylvania, and his office was in the 2nd National Bank Building there.

In the 1920 U.S. Census, Edward and Alice were renting a house on 5th Street in Pittsburgh. He was married to Alice, age 24. They had no children. They did have two live-in maids.[276] By 1930 they had prospered and were living in a house of their own at 6200 Woodland Road, Pittsburgh. Edward is noted as a surgeon. Their home was valued then at $100,000 (equivalent to almost 1.5 million in 2022 dollars). They appear to be childless.[277]

In 1940, the widower Edward was living on Woodland Road in Pittsburgh with his 70-year-old mother-in-law, Grace Hammond. Their house, worth $100,000 in 1930, was now valued a decade later at $50,000 ($880,000 in 2022 dollars), presumably because of the Depression.[278]

In May of 1941, he took out a marriage license to marry the widow Eleanor O. Dillon. She was born in Latrobe, Pennsylvania, in 1905. On their marriage license application it is stated that his former wife, Alice Hammond, had died in 1937.

Edward died January 2, 1966, in Pittsburgh after a long illness from complications of tuberculosis and a stroke. He was buried in the Homewood Cemetery in Pittsburgh in the same plot as his first wife, Alice Hammond Biddle.[279]

* * * * *

Poplawski, Private Stephen

Service number: 571437

Stephen Poplawski was born September 2, 1902, in Warsaw, Poland, to Melchier and Josephine (Sadowski) Poplawski.[280]

---

276. 1920 U.S. Census, Pittsburgh, Allegheny County, Pennsylvania.
277. 1930 U.S. Census, Pittsburgh, Allegheny County, Pennsylvania.
278. 1940 U.S. Census, Pittsburgh, Allegheny County, Pennsylvania.
279. https://www.findagrave.com/memorial/91025353/alice-r-pitcairn.
280. World War II draft cards, 1940–47, Stephen Poplawski.

Stephen was the youngest of four children. He had three known siblings: two sisters—Josephine (born about 1895) and Anna (born about 1900)—and a brother, Walter (born about 1896).

The 1920 U.S. Census showed Stephen's birth year as about 1900 and that he had emigrated to the United States in 1903 and was naturalized in 1908. But his birth year in that census was probably misstated for reasons shown below.

Leland Brown, the writer of this diary and letters, told his family about a fellow soldier who enlisted when he was below the enlistment age. Leland's story follows: A soldier of Field Hospital No. 33 wanted to enlist in the Army but was too young. The requirements for enlistment were to pass a physical examination and be both taller than 5'3" and between the ages of 18 and 38. Leland said that a soldier in his company was only 14 when he enlisted. The story was that this soldier said that he paid a "bum" (Leland's word) to swear that he was Stephen's father and that he was old enough to enlist. Unfortunately, the "bum" signed his own name and not that of Stephen's father and therefore Stephen was refused. He tried to enlist a second time and was accepted when his "father" lied about his age and signed Stephen's father's name and not this own.

Stephen enlisted at Columbus Barracks, Ohio, on November 23, 1917. At that time, he reported his age to be 18 years and two months.[281] When Stephen sailed to Europe with his company on May 26, 1918, he was four months shy of 19, according to his enlistment records. Army regulations stated that a soldier had to be 19 years old to be sent overseas. This fact was overlooked by the Army or perhaps that regulation had been changed by then.

The 1930 Census of Toledo, Ohio, recorded Stephen's birth year as 1903 (age 27 in 1930), which would have made him 14 when he enlisted on November 23, 1917. That census also shows that he was a veteran of World War I. It was therefore quite possible that Leland's story about a 14-year-old in his company referred to Stephen.

After his enlistment at the recruitment center at the Columbus Barracks, he was sent to Fort Oglethorpe, Georgia. There he received his early Army training at the Officers Training Camp. On December 1, 1917, he was attached to Field Hospital No. 33 at Camp Greene, North Carolina, for advanced training. Then, he sailed on May 26, 1918, to France with his outfit on the RMS *Melita*.

He was in Europe with Field Hospital No. 33 until he was transferred to Ambulance Company No. 28 of the 7th Division's Sanitary Train. He was honorably discharged on June 18, 1919. He was never promoted.

---

281. Ohio Soldiers in World War I, 1917–1918.

At some point after his honorable discharge Stephen reenlisted in the Army. In the U.S. Census for 1920 he is shown as a member of the Provisional Regiment of the 4th Division, which was stationed at Gary, Indiana. His rank was that of musician. No information about the Provisional Regiment was found. The 4th Division was deactivated at Camp Lewis, Washington, on September 21, 1921.

Leland said, at one point, that the same soldier who had lied about his age wanted to be transferred to the Army Air Corps. His transfer papers had to be approved by the company commander (probably Captain Fitzpatrick). His commander refused to approve the transfer saying, "I saved the Army one airplane."

Stephen traveled to Europe with the rest of his company on the RMS *Melita* in 1918 and returned on the SS *Minnesotan*.

For his service overseas, Stephen was eligible for the Victory Medal with the following clasps: Aisne-Marne; Saint-Mihiel, Meuse-Argonne, and the Defensive Sector.

About 1924, Stephen married Helen Sniegowski, who was born in Ohio to Polish parents.

In 1926 he was employed as a meat cutter. They lived at 1666 Belmont Avenue in Toledo, Ohio.[282]

The 1930 U.S. Census showed that Stephen rented their home at 1940 Dorr Street in Toledo, Ohio. Stephen and Helen had two sons: Melvin, born in 1925, and Robert, born in 1927. He was working in a meat market and was shown as a veteran of the World War. So, if he was born in 1903 (age 27 on the 1930 census) that would make him 14 when he enlisted in 1917. This alone is not enough to say that Stephen was the soldier that Leland was talking about. Yet, according to the 1930 census one can deduce that he was probably that same person.

In 1940 the Poplawskis were living on 902 Parkside Parkside Avenue in Toledo. They had a new daughter, Jane, age three. Melvin and Robert still lived with them, as did Helen's mother, Agnes Sniegowski, a widow. They owned their own home, which they valued at $4,000. Stephen was employed as the manager of a retail grocery store. Helen worked without pay as a clerk in that store.

When Stephen registered for the World War II Draft on February 15, 1942, he was working at the Kroger Grocery and Baking Co. on Dorr Street in Toledo. His draft card described him as being 5'11" tall, weighing 185 pounds, and having blue eyes and brown hair. The group photograph shown on the November 19, 1917, entry of this diary shows him as being

---

282. 1926 City Directory for Toledo, Ohio.

tall, but not the tallest of that group. Since he was about 15 when that photograph was taken, he might have added a few more inches to his height by 1942.

Stephen died April 10, 1962, in Toledo, Ohio, at age 60. His death certificate states his birth year was 1903, but many records suggest this is not entirely accurate. His World War II Draft card, which is filled out in his handwriting, clearly shows that he was born in 1902, which would mean that he was 15, not 14, when he enlisted. Life's little mysteries.

Rubley, Private First Class Erwin Morse

Service number: 571439

Erwin Rubley was born on August 1, 1895, in East Gilead, Indiana, to Charles Rubley and his wife, Zoe Morse Rubley.[283] Both of his parents were from Indiana. His father was a paper hanger.[284] In 1902 when Edwin was seven, the family moved to Michigan.

In 1910 they were living at 61 Inn Road in Battle Creek, Michigan, and by 1915 Erwin was working as a clerk in the Washington Avenue Pharmacy in Battle Creek.[285]

Erwin enlisted in the Medical Department of the Army on November 24, 1917.[286] It is assumed that he was sent to Fort Oglethorpe, Georgia, after his enlistment for his preliminary training. He was first mentioned in Leland's diary on January 16, 1918, when Rubley and several other privates were sent to the infirmary of the 16th Field Artillery at Camp Greene "to get some practical dope on hospital work." He was there for more than two weeks.

Rubley, along with most of Field Hospital No. 33, departed New York Harbor on May 27, 1918, on the RMS *Melita*. They landed at Liverpool, England, on June 7, 1918. He returned on the SS *Minnesotan* from Brest, France, on August 3, 1919. He was discharged at Camp Dix, New Jersey, on August 13, 1919. He was promoted to private first class while in France.[287]

While he was in France, waiting with his company to become part of the occupational forces in Germany, he wrote home the following to his father:

> A year ago yesterday I took the oath of a soldier, and one year later, on the same date, I entered German territory.

---

283. *Battle Creek Enquirer*, March 12, 1954, 26.
284. 1910 U.S. Census, Battle Creek, Michigan.
285. 1910, 1911, and 1915 City Directories for Battle Creek, Michigan.
286. *Battle Creek Enquirer*, March 12, 1954, 26.
287. *Battle Creek Enquirer*, March 12, 1954, 26.

I said I was In Germany, though it now belongs to France, but it has German customs and the German language is spoken, so it seems very much like Germany. We are here only for a few days and then we will go on into Germany. This Is the most wonderful part of Europe that I have seen so far.

We have seen as much of the fighting as any division over here and have done the best kind of work. We were in Auy Du Motien [Acy-en-Multien] when the drive started and stayed in until we had advanced as far as Fere En Tardinois. Then we were relieved and rested for three weeks: then we were in the St. Mihiel drive for a few days and went to the Argonne front just north of Verdun and were in action for a month. From there went to a town by the name of Villey Issay [Ville-Issey]. There we took life easy until we started out for occupation duty.

I had my own idea that the Germans would be a little cool, but they are fine so far, and I think that will continue so. I am now right in the heart of the Lorraine iron region. When it comes to machinery I have never seen anything to beat it.[288]

After the war, he came back to Battle Creek and continued as a pharmacist in partnership with Norman Freeman on Main Street. In Philadelphia, Erwin married Geraldine Isom on May 3, 1921.[289] She was born in 1893 to James Wiley Isom, a farmer, and Mary Effie Isom. The Isoms were all from Tennessee.

In September of 1925, Erwin sold both his interest in the West End Drug store and his house on High Street and moved to Houston, Texas.[290] There he continued in the drugstore business for eight years until they returned to Battle Creek. He worked for several drugstores before he opened his own store in 1939. It was across from the Post Cereal Factory at 15 Porter Street in Battle Creek. He managed that store for 15 years until his death.[291]

In 1928 while they were living in Texas, Erwin and Geraldine had their only child: Mary Evelyn Rubley. The Rubleys were in Houston. They owned their own home, which they valued at $5,000.[292]

In 1943 Erwin was accused of allowing boys to play a pinball machine in his store in Battle Creek. The police had secretly watched the boys play and questioned them when they left. They told the police that they had received two nickels when they had scored two free games on the pinball machine. A warrant was issued, and Rubley pleaded not guilty to the

---

288. *Battle Creek Enquirer*, January 5, 1919, 16.
289. Philadelphia, Pennsylvania, Marriage Index, 1885–1951.
290. *Battle Creek Enquirer*, September 1, 1925, 6.
291. *Battle Creek Enquirer*, March 12, 1954, 26.
292. U.S. Census, Houston, Texas.

charge. Three days later, however, he did plead guilty and paid a $50 fine. In his defense he said that he had returned to the boys the two nickels that they had put in the machine. After this incident he removed the pinball machine, possibly so there would be no further misunderstanding about the trafficking of nickels in his store.[293]

In 1954, Erwin was in ill health and went to Stockdale, Texas, where his sister-in-law and her husband lived. He was hoping the change might help him gain some strength. He died there from a heart condition on March 11 of that year. He was 58 years old.[294] His remains were returned to Battle Creek and buried in the Memorial Park Cemetery there.[295]

He was a member of the Retail Druggist Association, as well as a Mason and a Shriner.

His wife, Geraldine Isom Rubley, died on December 14, 1985. She was 92 years old.

* * * * *

Slay, Lieutenant Iris Joe

Service number: 156827

Iris Joe Slay was born in Many, Louisiana, on December 4, 1888, to James K. Slay, a farmer, and his wife, Cornelia Chandler. His parents were both born in Mississippi, as were his grandparents.

In 1900 Iris had three known siblings: Lucy Slay Calhoun, age 20, who was married to William Calhoun; Estella, age 19; and Ronald, age 10.[296, 297]

James Slay lost his wife and the children lost their mother when Cornelia died in 1904.

When Iris was about 20, he was appointed postmaster of Gulf, Mississippi. His appointment lasted for a little over 19 months until his post office was assimilated by the one in Richton, Mississippi.

The 1910 U.S. Census showed that Iris's 62-year-old father, James, was the head of the household. In that family was his divorced daughter, Lucy Slay Calhoun, and Lucy's 10-year-old daughter, Margaret. Lucy was keeping a boardinghouse, presumably in their home, as there were three boarders living at the same address. Other siblings of Lucy's were Estella, who at

---

293. *Battle Creek Enquirer*, March 22, 1943, 2.
294. *Battle Creek Enquirer*, March 12, 1954, 26.
295. Findagrave.com, Memorial Park Cemetery, Battle Creek, Michigan, Erwin M. Rubley.
296. 1900 U.S. Census, Marion, Mississippi.
297. World War I draft registration card (birthdate and place of birth).

29 was working as a trimmer in a millinery store; Ronald, 20, then in college; and Iris, 22, in medical school. They were living on Purvis Street in Purvis, Mississippi.[298]

In 1913, Iris graduated from the Memphis Hospital Medical College.[299]

On his World War I draft registration card dated June 5, 1917, he was shown to be of medium height and build with blue eyes and black hair. He was living and working in Vancleave, Mississippi.

On August 27, 1917, Iris enlisted in the Army.[300] Being a medical doctor, he was commissioned as a 1st lieutenant. He probably spent his preliminary army training at the Medical Officers Training Corps at Camp Greenleaf, Fort Oglethorpe, Georgia, before joining Field Hospital No. 33 at Camp Greene, North Carolina.

After the training of the soldiers at Camp Greene was completed, he sailed to Europe on the RMS *Melita* as the acting company commander of Field Hospital No. 33. This was because Major Fitzpatrick, the company commander, was already in France two weeks ahead of the company.[301]

After his service in France, he returned from Brest, France, on the USS *Leviathan*. He sailed on June 29, 1919, arriving at Hoboken, New Jersey, on July 5, 1919. He was discharged honorably from active duty at Camp Dix, New Jersey, three days later. His next of kin was his wife, Vera, living in DeRidder, Louisiana.[302]

In 1920 the Slay family were residing in their house with their three children: daughter Lollage (five) and two sons, Harold (three) and Iris Joe Jr. (one).[303]

In 1930 they were in Pineland Town, Texas, and they had added another daughter, Lucy, age nine. Iris was working as a doctor for the Temple Lumber Company, a large lumber company in that area. They rented their house for $14 a month and had a radio.[304]

By 1940, Iris and his wife, Vera, were divorced. Vera was living in Houston with her children: Harold, Iris Joe Jr., and Lucy. She was teaching in a public school. Her annual salary was $1,222. Harold and Iris Jr. were employed.

---

298. 1910 U.S. Census, Purvis, Mississippi.
299. *American Medical Association Directory*, 1918, 6th edition, A Registry of Legally Qualified Physicians of the United States.
300. Application for military headstone or marker.
301. Leland N. Brown diary.
302. U.S. Army Transport Service lists, 1910–1939.
303. 1920 U.S. Census, Liberty, Texas.
304. 1930 U.S. Census, Pineland, Texas.

Iris Sr. was living in Fostoria, Texas, with his new wife, Anna Jewel, 20 years his junior. She was the daughter of Eugene Francis and Mary Lea (Shoemaker) MacDonald. Anna was working as a nurse. Iris's annual income in 1940 was $3,540, and Anna's was $1,200.[305]

On January 15, 1941, he re-enlisted in the U.S. Army. In March 1941, he was transferred from Fort McIntosh, Texas, to the Panama Canal Zone. His rank was that of a major. He later saw duty at the Station Hospital at Fort Clark, Texas. The Fort Clark Hospital was a Black hospital under his command. The hospital had "a complement of 19 medical officers, 15 of whom are white." All of the nurses were Black.[306]

Iris retired from the Army on September 9, 1944, as a lieutenant colonel in the Medical Corps.

Vera Mae McLendon Slay, Iris's first wife, enlisted on May 6, 1944, at Fort Crockett, Galveston, Texas, in the Women's Army Corps as a private. Her enlistment record showed that she was a secondary school teacher, divorced and without dependents.[307]

Vera died on June 7, 1965, in Houston, Texas, at age 70 of a heart attack.[308] Her obituary mentioned her children: Iris J. Slay Jr., of Odessa, Texas, an Air Force major; Harold D. Slay of Paramariabo, Surinam, Dutch Guiana; Mrs. Lucy Love Willard of Houston; and Mrs. Lollage Deane of Beaverton, Oregon. Vera had been in school work for 51 years.[309] Vera was buried in the Forest Park Cemetery in Houston.[310]

Iris Joe Slay died on April 20, 1958, at age 69, probably in Purvis, Mississippi. He was buried in the Coal Town Cemetery in Purvis.[311]

Iris's second wife, Anna Jewell "Judy" McDonald Slay, died on November 5, 1999, at age 91. She is buried in the same cemetery as her parents, the Lone Star Cemetery in Pineland, Texas.[312]

Iris's grave marker shows him as Iris *Joe* Slay, while his son's grave marker is inscribed Iris *Joel* Slay, Jr.[313]

* * * * *

---

305. 1940 U.S. Census, Fosteria, Texas.
306. *Pittsburgh Courier*, July 17, 1943, 24.
307. World War II enlistment records, 1938–1946.
308. Texas Death Certificate #37422 for Vera Mae Slay.
309. *Liberty Vindicator*, Liberty, Texas, January 10, 1965, 3.
310. Texas Death Certificate #37422 for Vera Mae Slay.
311. Findagrave.com, Coal Town Cemetery, Purvis, Mississippi, Iris Joe Slay.
312. https://www.findagrave.com/memorial/13728771.
313. Findagrave.com, Cooke Memorial Cemetery, Liberty, Texas, Iris Joel Slay Jr.

Stewart, Cook Tom Lee

Service number: 571398

Tom Stewart was born on July 12, 1895, in Erastus, Jackson County, North Carolina[314] to Joseph W. and Mary Ann (Smith) Stewart. His parents were born in North Carolina, as were his grandparents.

In 1900 the Stewarts were living in Mountain Township in Jackson County, North Carolina. He had two older siblings, Wayne and Callie, and two younger sisters, Nancy and Lora.[315] The Stewarts owned their own farm.[316]

In 1917, when Tom Lee registered for the draft, he was described as short in height with dark hair and blue eyes.[317] He was working as a farmer.

On July 2, 1917, he enlisted in the Medical Department of the Army. It is likely that most, if not all, of the enlisted soldiers who were attached to Field Hospital No. 33 did their preliminary training at Camp Greenleaf, Fort Oglethorpe, Georgia, before going to Camp Greene, North Carolina, for their advanced medical and Army training.

While Tom was at Camp Greene, North Carolina, one of the medical officers, Lieutenant Iris Joe Slay, wrote to Tom's local newspaper the following:

> Dear Sir:
>
> This letter is in reference to Tom Lee Stuart [Stewart], from Mountain township, and I ask that you kindly publish it so that his friends and relatives may know what he is doing, and how fast he is making good. Tom Lee Stuart, whose father is Joseph Stuart, is 22 years old, enlisted in the Medical Department of the Army of Uncle Sam July 2nd, 1917, and has since given his service ungrudgingly and fully. He is now with Field Hospital No. 33, and is making good in every way. He has received recognition from his officers and has been made Private 1st Class, and was the only man in the entire detachment who received a pass to go home unconditionally. This pass was granted because of his faithful service. Every man in our unit has learned to admire Stewart, and we wouldn't give him up under any circumstances. The girls around his home would do an exceedingly wise thing if they managed to catch him on their string, as he would make all the fires early in the morning, and have a nice hot breakfast ready for them when they get up. Stuart will be home before long in his uniform, and will be shaking hands with his people and friends. We wish him the happiest time, and a safe return to us.
>
> Yours very truly, Iris J. Slay, 1st Lieut, M.R.C.[318]

---

314. World War I draft registration card, Jackson County, North Carolina, for Tom Lee Stewart.
315. 1910 U.S. Census.
316. 1900 U.S. Census.
317. World War I draft registration card, Jackson County, North Carolina, for Tom Lee Stewart.
318. *Jackson County Journal* (Sylvia, North Carolina), January 4, 1918, 5.

Stewart's pass to go home was from the December 23 to December 31, 1917.[319]

Sergeant Brown wrote about Stewart in his diary on March 1, 1918:

> Tom sure is a funny fellow. He was born in the country famous for its moonshine. That's how Tom came to join the army. He was driving a wagon load of "moonshine" down to town one day when the Revenue officers appeared on the scene. Tom left and left no trace. He doesn't even know what became of the "hoss" or the "licker."
>
> Last December the Captain gave Stewart a pass home. The railroad is 25 miles from his home and there was no way to go those 25 miles but the walk, so Stewart walked.
>
> Stewart never puts his shoes on in the morning when he first wakes up. It makes no difference what time he gets up or how cold it is, Stewart goes around his bare feet. Once he was asked why he did this he said, "The shoes are too cold and so are my feet. I wait until it gets warmer until I put my shoes on."
>
> One time he was going to box Gregg. Well, Stewart squared off, wound up his arm and cringo!!!!
>
> Gregg[320] was a half an hour coming around.

On March 1, 1918, Tom was appointed cook.[321]

While in Camp Greene, Sergeant Brown took a photograph of the cooks of Field Hospital No. 33. Perhaps Tom Lee is one of the cooks of Field Hospital No. 33 pictured on the next page.

On May 27, 1918, Tom sailed aboard the RMS *Melita* with Field Hospital No. 33 to Europe, landing in Liverpool, England. Several days later they crossed the English Channel to Le Havre, France.[322]

Tom returned to the United States aboard the *Giuseppe Verdi*, which sailed from Marseilles, France, on March 6, 1919. He was part of the St. Aignan Causal Company No. 1964, North Carolina.[323] He arrived at Jersey City, New Jersey, on March 2. He was then sent to Camp Merritt, New Jersey.[324]

In January of 1920, he was living with his parents on their farm, which they owned in Mountain Township, North Carolina. He was working as a laborer and as a teamster.[325]

---

319. Leland N. Brown diary.
320. Private First Class Herbert D. Gregg.
321. Leland N. Brown diary, March 2, 1918.
322. U.S. Army Transport Service passenger lists, 1910–1939.
323. Saint-Aignan was one of the several staging areas for casuals in France. It was at Saint-Aignan-des-Noyers, France. Casual companies are often organized according to where the soldier had lived before they entered the service; hence St. Aignan Casual Company, North Carolina.
324. U.S. Army Transport Service passenger lists, 1910–1939.
325. 1920 U.S. Census, Jackson County, Mountain, North Carolina.

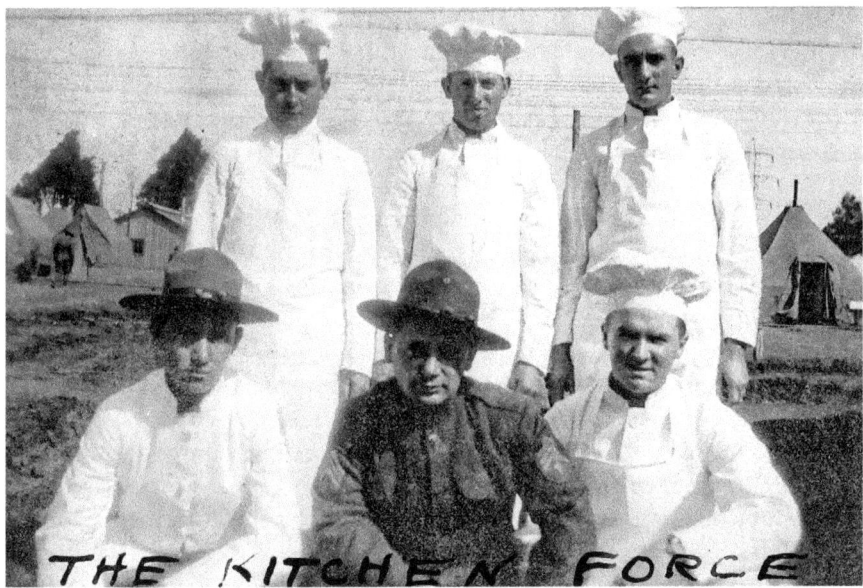

The Kitchen Force (photo album).

Toward the end of 1920, however, Tom became a patient at the U.S. Veterans Hospital in Augusta, Georgia, where he remained for almost thirteen years. He died there of tuberculosis at age 39, November 30, 1933. He never married.

He was buried in the Pine Creek Baptist Church Cemetery in Erastus, North Carolina.[326]

Wigington, Private James Walter

Service number: 571451

James Walter Wigington was born on October 30, 1899, in West Virginia to Samuel and Nancy Jane (Damron) Wigington. Samuel and Nancy had nine children, of which Walter was the eighth.[327]

His father died in 1902 and his widow, Nancy, remarried the next year to John D. Dalton. Nancy and John had one child, Lyndal Marie Dalton, who was born in 1906.

In 1910, when Arthur was nine, he was living with his brother Robert and his wife, Lizzie. In the same household were his mother, Nancy

---

326. Find a Grave Index
327. Virginia Harris, donginharr@ Ancestry.com.

Dalton, age 48, and his half sister, Marie Dalton, age three. Arthur's mother, Nancy, is shown as married, but her husband, John Dalton, was not listed with her in the 1910 census.

Robert Wigington was shown as a farmer working on his own account on a farm that he owned. That census shows that Nancy had had 10 children, of whom nine were still living. They were living in the Lincoln Magisterial District in West Virginia.[328]

When Walter was 18, he enlisted in the Medical Department of the Army at Fort Thomas, Kentucky, on November 19, 1917. His mother had died earlier that year. As with most of his Army outfit, he probably trained at Camp Greenleaf, Georgia, before coming to Camp Greene, North Carolina, where he received his advanced training with Field Hospital No. 33.

Around May 7, 1918, about 20 days before the company sailed to Europe, he and Private Enwright were reported A.W.O.L. and missing.[329]

Either he gave himself up or was arrested by the authorities, for on June 30, 1918, he sailed from Hoboken, New Jersey, to Europe on the SS *Siboney* as a private of Field Hospital No. 33.[330]

He was overseas with the Army for a little over 12 months. While he was in France, he participated in two offensives: Meuse-Argonne and Saint-Mihiel. He was not wounded or gassed, but he was hospitalized twice while in France, once for having influenza and again for scarlet fever.[331]

Although he was shown to be attached to Field Hospital No. 33 when he sailed to Europe, he was with the Medical Detachment of the 61st Infantry when he returned from France. He sailed on July 13, 1919, and arrived at New York on July 20 on the SS *Aquitania*. His sister, Mrs. Jennie Damron of Catlettsburg, Kentucky, was listed as his next of kin.[332]

James Walter Wigington was discharged from the Army on July 28, 1919, at Camp Taylor, Kentucky. He was not shown in the 1920 U.S. Census, but it is assumed that he was living in Catlettsburg.

In 1922 Walter married La Rosamond Mitchell in Catlettsburg. She was the daughter of James and Maggie Mitchell. James was a stonemason working for a railroad company.[333] Walter and La Rosamond had two daughters: Betty Ruth, born 1923, and Norma Virginia, born on January 23, 1925. In 1922 Walter and La Rosamond were divorced. He later stated during a neuropsychiatric exam that he had in 1936: "I made her get the

---

328. 1910 U.S. Census, Lincoln Magisterial District, Wayne County, West Virginia.
329. Leland N. Brown diary.
330. U.S. Army Transport Service, 1910–1939.
331. Virginia Harris, donginharr at Ancestry.com.
332. U.S. Army Transportation Service, 1910–1939.
333. 1910 U.S. Census, Catlettsburg, Kentucky.

divorce. I know I was going to do all the crooked stuff and I didn't want to pull my kids down."[334]

According to a family member, he was in the bootlegging business. He walked with a limp that resulted from being shot while burglarizing a warehouse.

In 1930 he was an inmate at the Kentucky State Reformatory in Franklin City, Kentucky.[335]

He died on October 12, 1951, in the Veterans Hospital in St. Cloud, Minnesota. There he had been an inmate for four years and three months. He died of pneumonia, which was brought on by a diffuse emphysema.[336] It was suspected that he had had Huntington's disease, which may have been a factor in his poor judgment that resulted in his criminal behavior.[337]

He was buried in the Catlettsburg Cemetery in Catlettsburg, Kentucky.[338] He was 51 years old.[339]

* * * * *

Wise, Mechanic Walter R.

Service number: 571402

Walter Wise was born in Pennsylvania on August 13, 1885, to Silas and Elizabeth Ann (Africa) Wise.[340] Both of his parents were natives of that state. By 1900 the family was living at 149 Maryland Avenue in Cumberland, Maryland. His father was a contractor-builder. Walter had five siblings: Myrtie E., born in 1874, a milliner; Edgar, born in 1878, a carpenter; Harry J., born in 1880, a railroad fireman; Bertha V., born in 1882; and Esther M., born in 1887. Walter was working as a postal clerk.[341]

About 1905, Walter married Iola E. Gregory from West Virginia. Their son, Glenson, was born about 1906 and their daughter, Milburn, in 1909.[342]

On November 25, 1917, Walter enlisted in the Army. At that time he was still living at 149 Maryland Avenue, Cumberland, Maryland. He probably received his basic training in the Medical Officers Training Corps at

---

334. Virginia Harris.
335. 1930 U.S. Census, Franklin City, Kentucky.
336. Minnesota Department of Health, Certificate of Death, James W. Wigington.
337. Virginia Harris.
338. U.S. Headstone Applications for Military Veterans, James W. Wigington.
339. Findagrave.com, Catlettsburg Cemetery, Catlettsburg, Kentucky, James Walter Wigington.
340. Ohio County Marriage Records for Licking County, Ohio, 1774–1993.
341. 1900 U.S. Census, Cumberland, Maryland.
342. 1910 U.S. Census, Cumberland, Maryland.

Camp Greenleaf, Georgia, before joining Field Hospital No. 33 at Camp Greene, North Carolina.

While with Field Hospital No. 33 he was promoted to private first class on January 14, 1918. When he shipped overseas on the RMS *Melita* on May 27, 1918, his rank was that of mechanic. His next of kin was his father, Silas Wise.[343] He was reduced to a private on February 14, 1919, and the next day he was transferred to Headquarters Company of the 77th Field Artillery. In that company his rank was that of a musician third class. During World War I he served in the following sectors: Aisne-Marne, Vesle, Toulon, Saint-Mihiel, and Meuse-Argonne.

He returned from Brest, France, to Hoboken, New Jersey, on July 29, 1919, on the USS *Tiger*.[344]

As some point during or before 1919, Iola and Walter were divorced. Iola was working as a laundry sorter in the Peerless Laundry Company in Cumberland. She was living at 204 North Mechanic Street there. The city directory for Cumberland shows her as living separately from Walter, but in that same directory, Walter is shown with Iola, and at the Mechanic Street address.

In the 1920 U.S. Census, Iola is at the same address with her 60-year-old mother, Emma Gregory, and Iola's two children, Glenson and Milburn. She is divorced and working as a laundry manager.

Walter, unmarried, lived with his father, and was a machinist with the Baltimore and Ohio Railroad.[345]

It appears Walter and Iola remarried at Newark, Ohio, on August 26, 1920. Their marriage license showed her as Mrs. Iola Wise, divorced, while Walter was shown as having been previously married.[346]

In 1930, Iola was living in East Cleveland, Ohio, working as a telephone operator for a laundry with her mother and two children: Milburn was a cashier, and Glenson worked as an odd job laborer. They did not have a radio. She was listed as a widow, and the assumption is that Walter had died.[347]

In 1940 Iola and her mother were living together, and she was still working the same laundry job.[348]

Iola died in Zanesville, Ohio, on February 10, 1972. She was 84. She is buried at Cedar Hill Cemetery in Newark, Ohio.[349]

* * * * *

---

343. U.S. Army Transport Service passenger Lists, 1910–1935.
344. U.S. Army Transport Service passenger Lists, 1910–1935.
345. 1920 U.S. Census, Cumberland, Maryland.
346. Ohio County Marriage Records for Licking County, Ohio, 1774–1993.
347. 1930 U.S. Census, East Cleveland, Ohio.
348. 1940 U.S. Census, East Cleveland, Ohio.
349. Findagrave.com.

Zink, Wagoner George Aloysius

Service number: 571403

George Zink was born on July 22, 1895, in Baltimore, Maryland, to Peter and Theresia (Ahles) Zink. Both Theresia and Peter were born in Maryland to parents of German ancestry. George's father, Peter, was employed by the Baltimore and Ohio Railroad as a bricklayer. By 1910 George had an older sister, Amalia, and five younger brothers: Herman, Frank, William, Bernard, and Edward. They were living at 218 North Wolfe Street with his mother's father, George Ahles. At age 15, George Zink worked as an office boy for a newspaper.[350] He did not attend school after the fifth grade.

On June 5, 1917, when George registered for the draft, he was described as having a medium height and build, dark hair, and brown eyes. At that time, he was living on Streeper Street in Baltimore and working as a printer for the Price Company at 23 South Calvert Street in that city. He claimed to be supporting his mother and his two brothers and sister—all under 12 years of age.[351]

In 1914 when George was 19, his father died.[352]

George enlisted in the Army on June 22, 1917. He then went to

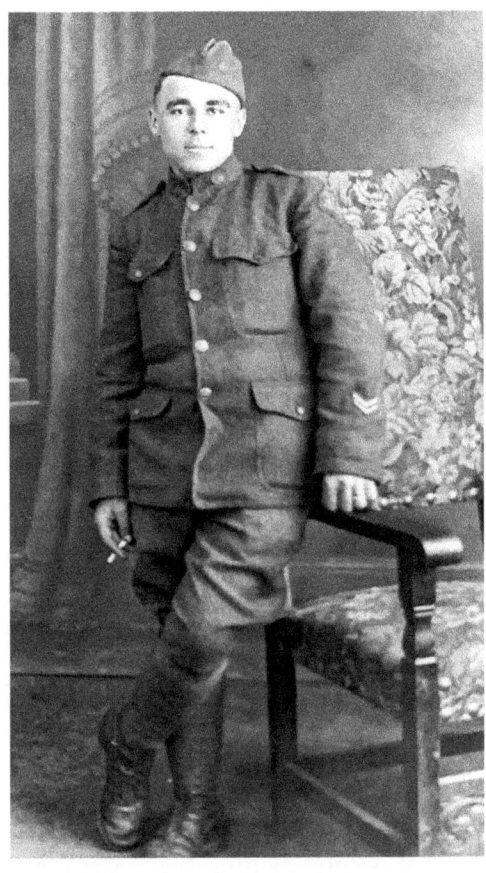

Private George Zink in Europe. On his left sleeve are two stripes. Each stripe denotes six months of overseas service (courtesy of Jo Ann Duprey).

---

350. 1910 U.S. Census, Baltimore, Maryland.
351. World War I draft registration card.
352. Findagrave.com, Holy Redeemer Cemetery, Baltimore, Maryland.

Officers Training Camp at Fort Oglethorpe, Georgia, where he was attached to the Regimental Hospital No. 54 before coming to Camp Greene, North Carolina. There he was attached to Field Hospital No. 33.[353]

He was promoted to private first class on January 14, 1918. On May 27, 1918, George sailed from Hoboken, New Jersey, to Europe with Field Hospital No. 33 on the RMS *Melita*. While in Europe on August 13, 1918, his rank was reduced to private.

He returned on the SS *Minnesotan* and arrived in Philadelphia on August 3, 1919. He was honorably discharged at Camp Dix, New Jersey, three days later.[354]

While in service with Field Hospital No. 33 in France, he was active in the following campaigns: Aisne-Marne, Vesle Sector, Toulon Sector, Saint-Mihiel, and Meuse-Argonne.[355]

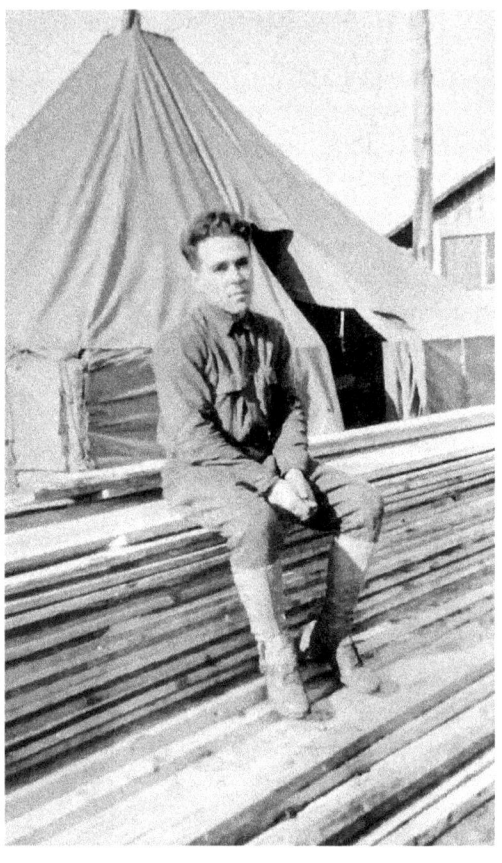

Private George Zink at Camp Greene, North Carolina, 1917 (courtesy of Jo Ann Duprey).

In 1920, George returned to Baltimore and moved into the house on Streeper Street where he had previously lived. On the census of that year, in addition to his mother, six of George's siblings were living with him: Frank, William, Bernard, Edward, Marie, and the widow Amalia (Zink) Ridgley and her three children. George was working as a printer in a print shop.

Soon after returning home, George married Hilda M. Stallings. Hilda was the daughter of George and Sadie Stallings. They had one child,

---

353. Maryland Military Men, 1917–1918.
354. Maryland Military Men, 1917–1918.
355. Maryland Military Men, 1917–1918.

George Zink, Jr., born August 25, 1921.[356] In the 1922 City Directory for Baltimore, George and Hilda were living at 719 Carlswell Street in Baltimore. He was working in a press foundry. By 1924 they moved to 712 North Streeper Street. In 1930 Hilda was no longer living with them. She was a patient in the Springfield State Hospital in Sykesville, Maryland.

In 1930 his family was at the 712 Streeper Street property, which they owned. His mother, Theresia, was the head of the family. George and three of his siblings lived there too: William, Edward, and Marie, along with George's son, George Jr. The census showed that George was married about 1920, but his wife was not listed. Two of his brothers were out of work, which was not surprising as this was the height of the Great Depression. The other two siblings, Edward and Marie, were working in a grocery store. George was employed as a printer. The yearly income for the household was $2,800.[357] In 1940 the family—George; his mother, Theresia; and his son, George Jr.—was residing at 2821 Biddle Street in Baltimore, which they rented for $24 month. George was working as a book printer. His yearly income was $1,200.[358]

In 1942 George was working for the Rustless Iron & Steel Company in Baltimore. He was 5'10" tall, weighed 190 pounds, and had blue eyes, brown hair, and a ruddy complexion.[359]

His mother, Theresia, died on May 23, 1947, in Baltimore. At the time of her death, she was living at the North Streeper Street house.[360]

George died on January 3, 1965, while residing at 3112 Baybrier Road in Baltimore. His obituary states that he was survived by his wife, Marie Moore Zink, and his children: George A. Jr., Thomas A., Daniel R., Bernard W., and Mrs. Marie Jones.

He was buried in Moorland Memorial Park in Baltimore. He was 69 years old.[361]

George's first wife, Hilda Marie Stallings Zink, died in January 1974 at the Springfield State Hospital in Sykesville, Maryland, where she was a patient.[362] Because of George's strong belief that marriage was dissolved only by death, he never divorced Hilda.

* * * * *

---

356. From Ancestry.com, Jo Ann Zink Duprey.
357. 1930 U.S. Census, Baltimore City, Maryland.
358. 1940 U.S. Census, Baltimore City, Maryland.
359. World War II draft registration card for George Aloysius Zink.
360. *The Evening Sun* (Baltimore, Maryland), May 26, 1947, 31.
361. *Baltimore Sun*, January 3, 1965, 38.
362. Springfield Hospital Center, Sykesville, Maryland, Medical Records.

Zipse, Private First Class Richard Julius

Service number unknown

Private Richard Zipse was born in November 1898 in New York to Ernst (Ernest) and Maggie (Margaret) Ruttger Zipse. Ernest emigrated to the United States in 1881 from Germany. Richard's mother was born in New York to German parents. The family was living at 213 East 89th Street in Manhattan. Ernest was a bartender in a hotel.[363]

Richard had several brothers and sisters. By 1910 the family had moved to 372 7th Street in Brooklyn. They owned their home, which was mortgaged.

In 1915 Richard was in school and his family lived in the same house on 7th Street. His older brother Arthur was working as draftsman, and his sister Amelia was a stenographer.

Richard enlisted in the Regular Army at Fort Slocum, New York, on September 27, 1917.[364] He probably did his basic training at Fort Oglethorpe in Georgia before joining Field Hospital No. 33 at Camp Greene, North Carolina.

He was promoted to private first class on January 16, 1918.[365]

He did not serve overseas as he was honorably discharged on March 7, 1918, before his unit was sent to France. The cause of his discharge was a "SCD: service connected disability."[366] Sergeant Brown mentions him in his diary as swaying and unable to stand still, which was the cause of his discharge.

In 1925 he was still living with his parents at 467 8th Street in Brooklyn along with his sisters Amelia, Edna, and Margaret and his brother Edwin. Both he and Amelia were working as stenographers; Margaret was in business school, and Edwin was a student in college.[367]

In 1930 Richard was unmarried and living at 467 8th Street in Brooklyn with his parents and two sisters. He was working as a stenographer in an electrical office.[368]

On March 7, 1933, Richard Zipse died in Los Angeles.[369] His remains were sent to Brooklyn.[370] He was buried in the Green-Wood Cemetery in Brooklyn on March 16, 1933.[371] He was 34 years old.

Jean Cherfils was a French soldier whom Sergeant Brown met at Bourget when he first came to France, and they kept in touch afterwards.

---

363. 1905 New York State Census.
364. New York Abstracts of World War I Service 1917–1919.
365. Leland N. Brown diary.
366. New York Abstracts of World War I Service 1917–1919.
367. 1905 New York State Census.
368. 1930 U.S. Census.
369. *Brooklyn Daily Eagle*, March 12, 1933, 20.
370. *Los Angeles Times*, March 11, 1933, 10.
371. Green-Wood Cemetery, Brooklyn, New York, Records.

The Personnel of Field Hospital No. 33

A transcription of Jean Cherfils's postcard:

Dear friend,
August 12th '18

    I take pleasure in answering to you. I received your letter from August 2nd this morning, the first I have in hands since I saw you at Bourget two months ago I expect. I am very sorry not having seen you when I was wounded. Then who says you I was hurt? Perhaps the American soldier who carried [me] over from the lines tell the French ambulance.

    I am now at Paris in a hospital where we are very well nursed. The surgeon has esctracted [sic] the burst of the shell [shrapnel] that I had in my thigh. I must keep [to] bed but I shall be cured soon and I shall have a good convalescence at Rouen before to come back on the front. Parisians and all the French people are fond of your army. Did you see them to welcome you on last July 4th (your Independence Day). I shall send you my photo in the next letter. Do you think if I send you a packet of jams, cakes, sweet meats you shall receive it?? I did not pay postage for your letter I expect it is the same for the [as for] mine.

    Good luck dear friend. If you come to Rouen dont forget to go home [come here] where you will be well come. Remembrance from a young French soldier,
    Answer me at Rouen 14 Rue Walter
    Seine Inférieure

    Sincerely yours,
    Jean Cherfils

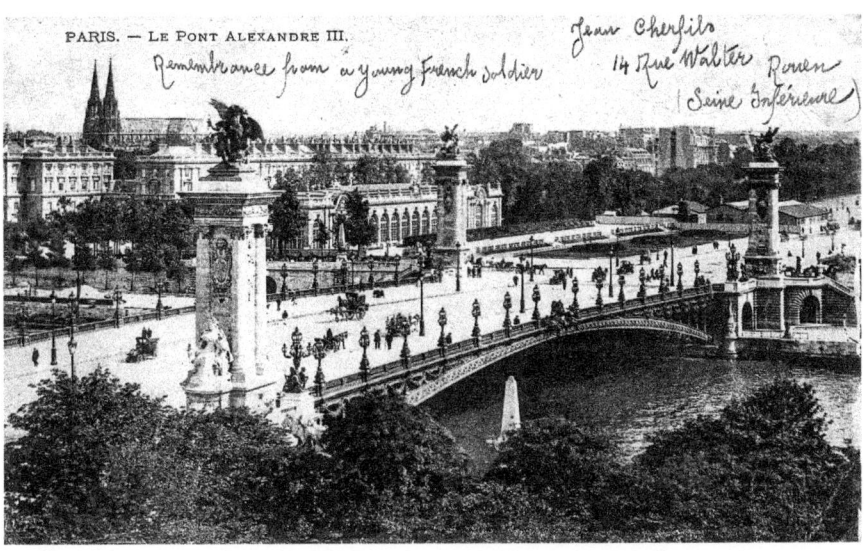

A postcard Sergeant Brown received from Jean Cherfils, a French soldier whom he met on a railroad siding at Le Bourget when he first landed in France. Their meeting is mentioned in the diary entry of June 15, 1918. Le Bourget is a small town near Paris just east of Saint-Denis. Le Bourget is shown on the map before his 2 p.m. diary entry of July 16, 1918.

Appendix B

Jean Adolphe Cherfils was born on November 25, 1898, in Rouen, France, to Adolphe Gaston Constant Cherfils and Marie Marguerite Alexandrine Peltier.

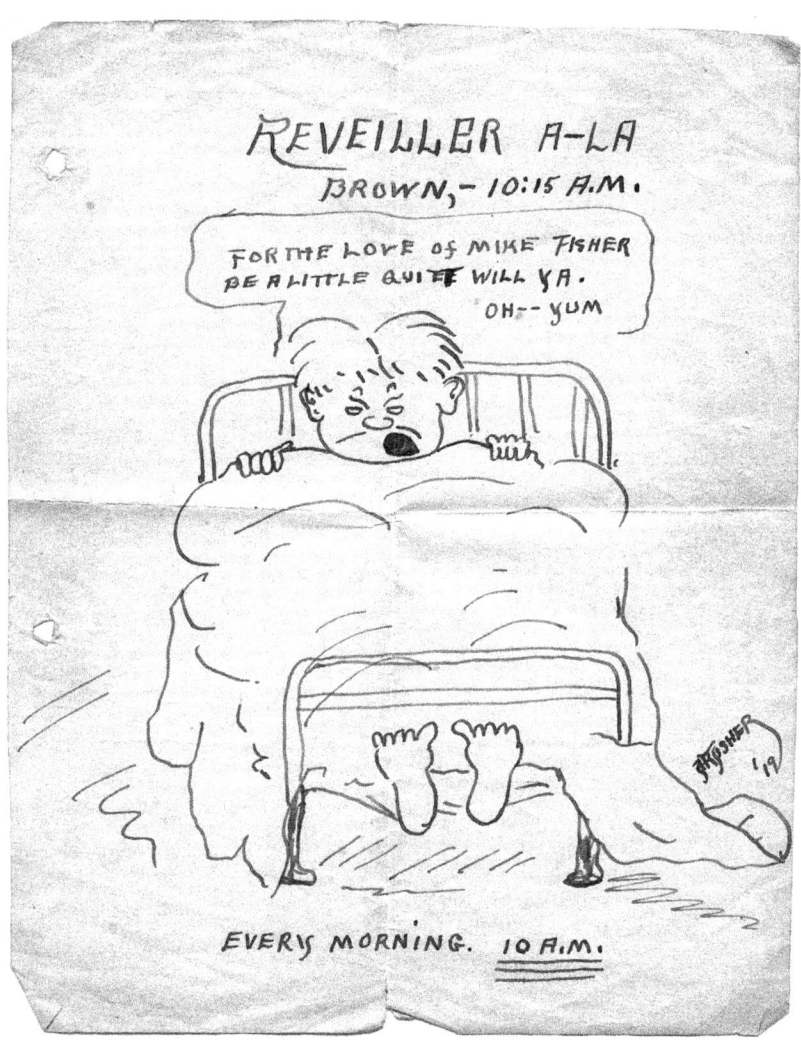

Two cartoons by 1st Sergeant Arthur Fisher, Sergeant Brown's fellow soldier throughout his enlistment and his housemate while they were part of the occupation in Germany. They came up through the ranks together from privates to sergeants first class. The cartoons were not attached to the diary but were among loose papers that accompanied it. Fisher is mentioned nine times in Brown's diary. On September 30, 1918, when Leland was gassed, Fisher looked after Sergeant Brown in the evacuation ward of Field Hospital No. 33.

The Personnel of Field Hospital No. 33

He was a high school student living at 14 Rue Walter in Rouen when he enlisted. He was described as having dark blond hair, brown eyes, an oval face, and an uplifted, erect nose. He was one meter 66 centimeters tall (about 5'5") with light burns on his chest.

He enlisted on April 19, 1917, as a soldier second class. He advanced

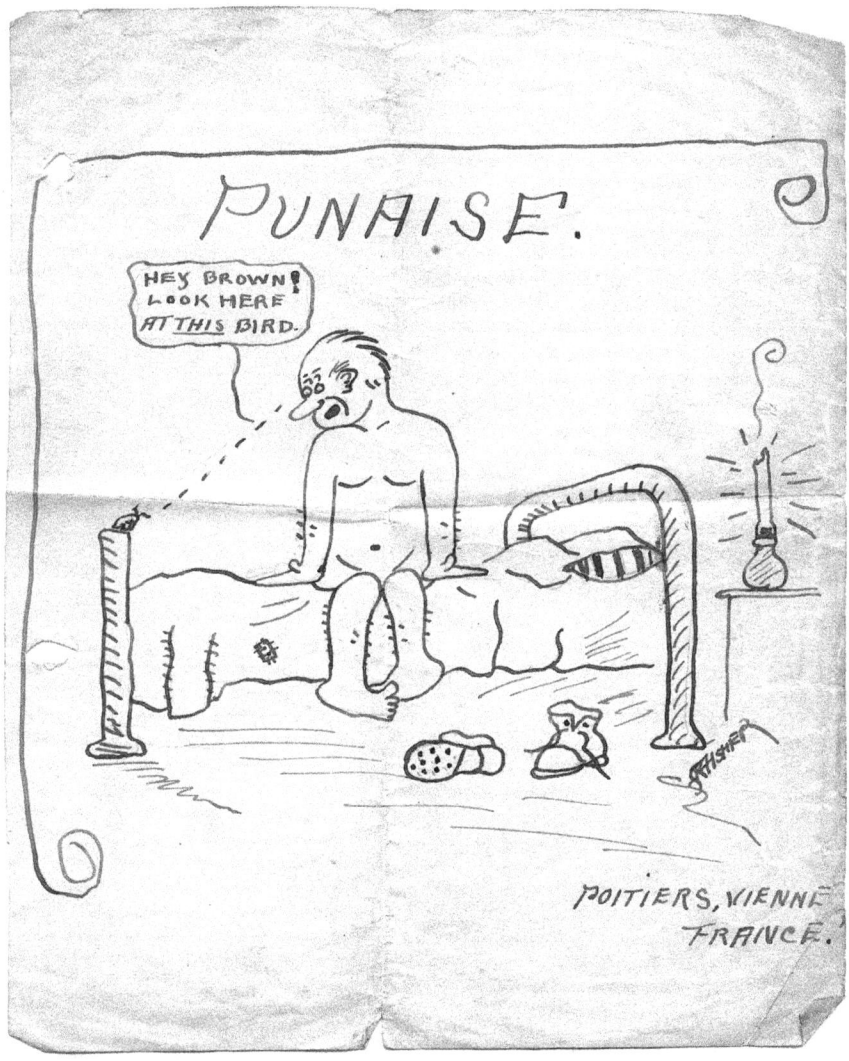

The "*Punaise*" cartoon is set in Poitiers, France, which suggests that Fisher had accompanied Sergeant Brown there and was taking classes at the University of Poitiers as well. The implication is that Brown is a late sleeper, which is often referred to in the diary and is reinforced in the drawing.

to sergeant on March 20, 1919. He was in the regular French army until October 23, 1919, and later in the reserves until 1939.

He was wounded in his right knee by artillery shrapnel near Dormans, France, on July 18, 1918, during the Battle of the Marne. He awarded the Croix de Guerre medal with a bronze star. There is no indication that Sergeant Brown and Jean Cherfils ever met again after their first encounter at Le Bourget on June 14, 1918.

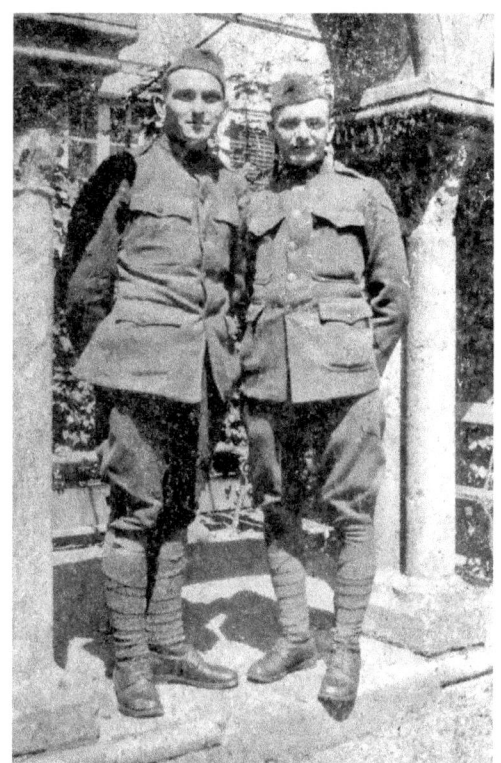

Sergeant Brown (on left) with a friend, who is possibly 1st Sergeant Arthur Fisher. This photograph was probably taken in Poitiers, France, while Fisher and Brown were studying at the university there (photo album).

Bibliography

American Medical Directory, 6th ed. Chicago: American Medical Association, 1918.
Bach, Christian Albert, and Henry Noble Hall. *The Fourth Division: Its Services and Achievements in the World War*. Country Life Publishers, 1920.
Davis, Evans. *The First World War*. Chicago: Contemporary Books, 2004.
Gilbert, Martin. *The First World War: A Complete History*. New York: Henry Holt and Company, 1994.
Gray, Randel, with Christopher Argyle. *Chronicle of the First World War, Volume II: 1917–1921*. Oxford, UK: Facts of File, Ltd, 1991.
Howard, Michael. *The First World War*. New York: Oxford University Press, 2002.
Keegan, John. *The First World War*. New York: Alfred A. Knopf, 1999.
Lynch, Charles, Frank W. Weed, and Loy McAfee, eds. *The Medical Department of the United States Army in the World War*. Washington, D.C.: U.S. Army Surgeon General's Office, 1923–29. https://achh.army.mil/history/book-wwi-seriesbklst.
Lynch, Charles, Joseph H. Ford, and Frank W. Weed. *Field Operations. The Medical Department of the United States in the World War*, Volume VIII. Washington, D.C.: Government Printing Office, 1925.
"Medicine in the First World War." The University of Kansas Medical Center. https://www.kumc.edu/school-of-medicine/academics/departments/history-and-philosophy-of-medicine/archives/wwi.html.
Mitchell, Miriam Grace, and Edward Spaulding Perzel. *Echo of the Bugle Call: Charlotte's Role in World War I*. Charlotte, NC: Dowd House Preservation Committee Citizens for Preservation Inc., 1979.
National Library of Medicine. https://www.nlm.nih.gov/.
Simonds, Frank H. *History of the World War*, Vol. V. Garden City, NY: Doubleday, Page & Company, 1920.
Tucker, Spencer C., ed. *The European Powers in the First World War: An Encyclopedia*. New York: Garland Publishing Co., 1966.
United States Department of State, Office of the Historian. "Milestones in the History of U.S. Foreign Relations, 1914–1920: World War One and the Wilsonian Diplomacy." https://history.state.gov/milestones/1914-1920.

Index

Acy-en-Multien, France 56
Adragna, Private Marco 150
American hospital train 103–4
Army Nurse Corps 125
Arrowsmith, Private Ernest Henry 152
artwork noted 57
aviators 126

Barkman, Private Frank 154
Battle of Belleau Wood 69–70
Battle of the Argonne Forest *see* Meuse-Argonne Offensive
Battle of the Marne 82, 224
Battleship *Celtic* 42
Battleship *New Hampshire* 42
Beaune, Germany 137
Biddle, Private John Young 22, 150
Borden, Premier Robert Laird 40, 43
Bowman, Sergeant Jess 23, 87, 158
Brest, France 137, 140
Bulcy, France 113
Burt, James 114
burying the dead 66, 67, 69, 70

Cameron, Major General George 128
Camp Dix, New Jersey 137
Camp Greene, North Carolina 139, 147–9
Camp Greenleaf, Fort Oglethorpe, Georgia 9, 11, 139, 145–7, 149
Camp Merritt, New Jersey 38, 40
casualties 61, 89, 138
Château de la Forêt, France 70, 71
Château Montebise *see* Pierre Levee, France
Château-Thierry, France 82–3, 94, 115
Cherfils, Jean 221–4
conditions (Army hospital) 80, 86, 97
Cooper, Corporal Raymond Johnson 160
Cuisy, France 85, 93, 99, 102, 109
Curran, Captain George Lally 106, 111, 115, 123, 125, 162

Daniel, Private First Class Guy Rogers 164
Davis, Private 126
De Benneville, Sergeant 1st Class (Bert) Bell 121
Delo, Private Carmen Chester 166
Dick, Lieutenant Walter 150, 168
Dick, Private Albert 169

Eberle, Wagoner Fred P. 138, 171
English soldiers 45
Enwright, Private Philip Joseph 150, 172
Épaux-Bézu, France 2, 63, 69–71, 112

family (of Sergeant Brown) 7, 37, 39, 55, 78, 87, 94, 100, 122, 142–3
Fère-en Tardenois, France 2, 69–70, 73, 111
Fick, Major 111, 112
field hospitals 9, 10, 19, 21, 33, 63–4, 75, 80, 86, 94
Fisher, Sergeant First Class Arthur 103, 128, 130, 173, 222–3
Fitzpatrick, Major Francis Percival 175
Fourth Division 31, 131–5
French soldiers 77, 79

Garden, Private John 21
gas 93, 95; gas hospital 93; gas mask 46; gas poisoning experience 102–4
Germans 52, 53, 54, 59, 61, 65, 66, 99
Germans' battle conditions 34, 66–9, 89
Green, Cook Stephen 21
Grimer, Private 21
Grimm, Private 21

Hall, Lieutenant 21
Harding, George 92
Haudainville, France 80, 124
Hersey, General M.L. 131
Hind, Sergeant Edward Wellyn, Jr. 177
Hodsdon, Sergeant First Class Merle 91, 179

Index

Hoeber, Frank 130
Holland, Harry 7, 95, 124, 142
Huid, Sergeant Eddie 121

illnesses among troops 21, 23, 28, 77, 114, 213
impressions of England 44–5, 47
impressions of France 47, 48, 49, 56, 58, 75–7, 82, 108–9, 112

Johnson, First Lieutenant Leighton 180
Jongbloed, Sergeant Auke "Andrew" 182

Kaiser, abdication of 97
Kaisersesch, Germany 128, 135
Kerensky, Alexander 107
Kersky, Private Philip 23–4
King, Sergeant Lawrence 22, 151, 185
Kitchener, Lord 107

La Charité, France 95–7, 123
Lemmes, France 80, 83, 85
Liffol-le-Petit, France 74, 85
Lighthall, Alma, R.N. 111
Lista, Private First Class Peter 186
Lombard, Sergeant First Class Steven 150, 188
Lynch, Captain 97

Mannas, Private Charles 190
maps: Allied marches in September 1918 in eastern France 84; American area of occupation Dec. 21, 1918 133; American troops travel, June-July 1918 72; eastern France (Vitry to Culsy) 84; marches along the Marne, August 1918 71; route between Toul and Kaisersech 132
Marian (girlfriend) 5, 6, 38, 73, 78, 106, 121, 129, 142
McDonnell, Private Thomas Francis 191
Meaux, France 60, 61, 71, 72, 82, 100
medals 140–2
RMS *Melita* 40, 43
Mesves, France 85, 99, 101, 110–125
Metz, Germany 79, 89, 97, 128, 132
Meuse-Argonne Offensive 79, 88–93
SS *Minnesotan* 137
Mitchell, Colonel "Billy" 79
Model T Ford ambulance 59, 60
Monahan, Corporal Joseph 14
Mullaney, Private James 196

Neufchâteau, France 82
Nevers, France 114
Nice, France 112, 115
Nyakowski, Private Frank J. 21

Ollig, Käthe 129–30

Paquette, Private 198–9
Patton, Lieutenant Colonel George 79
Pennsylvania National Guard 126
Pershing, General John J. 53, 55, 75, 78, 79, 135–7
Philadelphia College of Pharmacy 7
Phillips, Major John Charles 106, 130, 199
Pierre-Levée, France 48
Pitcairn, Captain Edward 202
Plummer, Captain 111, 113, 114
Poplawski, Private Stephen 203
Pouilly, France 109

railroad: French 74, 79, 96–7; German 89; hospital train 103–4
Rambluzin 79, 80, 83, 85
recreation and entertainment for troops 30–1, 35–6, 43
Ring, Lieutenant 21, 23
Roche, Ethel Emily 165
Roosevelt, Lieutenant Quentin 94
Rubley, Private First Class Erwin 150, 206

Saint-Mihiel offensive 78–80, 88, 99
Saint-Quentin battle 33, 34
Sanitary Train 9
Second Battle of the Marne 61, 75, 82
Shearer, Private LeRoy 20, 21, 37, 150, 173
Sivry-la-Perche, France 80, 84–94, 99, 102
Skinner, William Burdette "Bert" 117
Slay, Lieutenant Iris Joe 208
Soldo, Private Charles J. 20–22
Stewart, Cook Tom 211
Szypkowski, Lieutenant 110

Thorne, Eddie 122, 124
tobacco 42, 43, 75
Toul, France 126, 132
treatment of prisoners of war 54, 55

University of Poitiers 137

Vaux-Lorey, France 76
Vavincourt, France 78
Verdun, France 91, 124
Vitry-le-François, France 82

Walters, Sergeant 91, 106, 110
Wigington, Private James Walter 150, 213
Wise, Mechanic Walter R. 215

Zinc, Wagoner George 217
Zipse, Private First Class Richard 220

www.ingramcontent.com/pod-product-compliance
Ingram Content Group UK Ltd.
Pitfield, Milton Keynes, MK11 3LW, UK
UKHW041944140426
5217IPUK00014B/654